Surgical Procedures in Primary Care

Surgical Procedures in Primary Care *An Illustrated Guide*

MICHAEL BULL
and
PETER GARDINER

OXFORD UNIVERSITY PRESS
Oxford   New York   Tokyo
1995

Oxford University Press, Walton Street, Oxford OX2 6DP

Oxford New York
Athens Auckland Bangkok Bombay
Calcutta Cape Town Dar es Salaam Delhi
Florence Hong Kong Istanbul Karachi
Kuala Lumpur Madras Madrid Melbourne
Mexico City Nairobi Paris Singapore
Taipei Tokyo Toronto
and associated companies in
Berlin Ibadan

Oxford is a trade mark of Oxford University Press

Published in the United States
by Oxford University Press Inc., New York

A catalogue record for this book is available from the British Library

Library of Congress Cataloging in Publication Data
Bull, M. J. V.
Surgical procedures in primary care: an illustrated guide/
M. J. V. Bull; illustrated by Peter Gardiner.
Includes bibliographical references and index.
1. Surgery, Minor. 1. Title.
[DNLM: 1. Surgery, Minor—methods—handbooks. 2. Family Practice—
Great Britain—handbooks. WO 39 B935s 1994]
RD111.B85   1994   617'.024—dc20   93—45783

ISBN 0 19 262458 X

Typeset by Cambrian Typesetters Frimley, Surrey
Printed in Hong Kong

To Ida and Sharon

Preface

The New Contract for general practice in the National Health Service introduced in 1990 in the United Kingdom included, amongst many other innovations, payment on a sessional basis for minor surgical procedures undertaken by family doctors. Until this point, minor surgery had been a somewhat neglected area within the Health Service, largely on account of the time required and expenses associated with an activity offering no return other than personal satisfaction for the doctor and convenience for the patient. However, now that the service is recognized by statutory remuneration, there has been a reawakening of interest in skills that may have grown rusty since post-registration days in the casualty department or operating theatre. Furthermore, with an ever-widening clinical curriculum for medical students and with the accent in vocational training increasingly orientated towards behavioural and holistic medicine, it is perhaps appropriate to redress the balance with the publication of a volume directed towards the actual practicalities of minor surgery.

Although the basic principles of surgical practice in any setting are addressed in the preliminary chapters, this handbook is purposely aligned to the categories of procedures which might now be undertaken by general practitioners in the United Kingdom and which are listed in Paragraph 42, Schedule 1, of the National Health Service General Medical Services Statement of Fees and Allowances (the Red Book). Whilst it is to be hoped that the great majority of procedures described herein will qualify for remuneration, clinical description of any procedure in this book does not of itself imply that such an operation is automatically an allowable procedure for payment under the terms of the general practitioner minor surgery scheme.

For the benefit of practitioners unfamiliar with some of the techniques illustrated, the format for each procedure has been standardized: after a brief introduction, the equipment is listed and the method then illustrated in a sequential series of diagrams. This style of presentation was devised by Peter Gardiner and, for the most part, the procedures were photographed from real-life cases and converted to art work by him. Many have already been published in the 'Practical Procedures' series in the weekly medical magazine *Doctor* and we are indebted to the editor of that journal for permission to reproduce them. We appreciate, of course, that there are alternative techniques for many of the operations illustrated and some readers may consider that their own approach to a problem has advantages over those recommended here. Nevertheless, so far as the general practitioner author is concerned, the methods described have proved satisfactory in over 35 years in practice and, thus, may be recommended with confidence to fellow practitioners.

In principle, we believe that it is of paramount importance that only procedures which are unquestionably safe for the patient are undertaken by general practitioners. This proviso requires that the conditions to be treated must be readily accessible and are those that can be managed **without** the need for general anaesthesia, a policy that is clearly manifest in the regulations. Furthermore, we believe that the procedures illustrated will be possible in most practice premises nowadays with some nursing assistance and without the need for highly sophisticated operating theatre furniture or equipment. We pay attention to the question of selection and sterilization of instruments, aseptic technique, and aftercare. Medico-legal aspects are briefly addressed and references and sources of further information are detailed at the end of each chapter. Ultimately, of course, success in the field of minor surgery requires a sufficient degree of skill on the part of the operator and it is this aspect that our book primarily seeks to address. As in any field of medicine, confidence and expertise will only develop with time and we urge any reader who remains uncertain after perusing our text and illustrations to take advice from an experienced colleague as well.

1994   M. J. V. B.
P. G.

Acknowledgements

We are indebted to the editor of the weekly medical magazine *Doctor* for permission to reproduce the procedures originally published by him and to Dr Donal Hynes, Dr Chris Kenyon, and Dr Tim Sonnex who also contributed to that series. We are grateful to Drs Kate Allsopp and Mary-Lou Nesbitt (Medical Defence Union Ltd) for advice on medico-legal aspects of minor surgery and to Dr Dick Mayon-White (Department of Community Medicine, Oxford University) for help with occupational health problems. Dr Tom Jones (Oxfordshire Family Health Services Authority) assisted with administrative queries associated with the New Contract. Mr Michael Greenhall (John Radcliffe Hospital, Oxford) advised on sclerotherapy and Dr John Wilkinson (The Chiltern Hospital, Great Missenden) allowed us to reproduce the patient information leaflet (Chapter 4). We are also obliged to Howard Griffiths (editor, *Pulse* magazine) for permission to reproduce Figs 1.1 and 1.2, to Dr David Morgan (Head of Scientific Affairs, British Medical Association) for Table 1.2, to Dr R. T. Mayon-White for Table 2.1, Dr G. A. J. Ayliffe for Fig. 2.1, and Dr D. A. Kelly for Fig. 3.1. Our thanks are also due to our many patients who permitted procedures to be photographed prior to conversion to artwork, to the treatment room sisters at St Bartholomew's Medical Centre, Oxford, for their tolerant cooperation, and, finally, to one of the author's small grandsons for permitting the hypothetical removal of foreign bodies from various orifices.

Contents

1 Premises, instruments, and equipment

Good work and job satisfaction in any profession require satisfactory premises and appropriate equipment and this is especially the case where a service for minor surgery is to be provided in general medical practice. Although improvisation is sometimes necessary, high quality work on a continuing basis is greatly facilitated by satisfactory accommodation and the availability of the necessary instruments and equipment.

Design of premises for minor surgery

Nowadays, as GPs increasingly work from purpose-built premises, an area is usually set aside for practical treatment by nurses and this section will often include provision for minor operations. Of course, many simple surgical procedures can be undertaken in rooms normally used for other purposes, for example, general treatment areas, examination rooms, or even in the consulting room. However, when direct payment of rent and rates is being claimed under current NHS regulations, the minimum standards specified in the *Statement of fees and allowances* (SFA) (NHS General Medical Services 1990) require that (Paragraph 51.10 (h)) 'where the premises are used for minor surgery, a suitable room and equipment for the procedures for which the room and equipment is used' should be provided.

For doctors in larger practices contemplating new building or conversion of existing premises, the following points may offer some guidance for the design of a combined nursing treatment room and minor surgery area. The basic accommodation should comprise

(1) subwaiting area for patients;
(2) specimen collection facilities;
(3) clean preparation and storage area;
(4) nurse treatment area;
(5) minor surgery theatre;
(6) clinical waste disposal facilities.

A room-relationship diagram for planners is shown in Fig. 1.1 and the new layout for a conversion made some years ago in an existing health centre is shown as an example in Fig. 1.2. When architects are employed in the design of new buildings it is important that they are conversant with design requirements for medical practice and have experience in this particular field. Over elaboration should be avoided, for example, whilst good ventilation and ease of cleaning are important, antistatic floors are rarely necessary unless inhalational anaesthesia is contemplated. Design guides published over 20 years ago (see References) still form a good basis for planning new premises and an up-to-date résumé of NHS regulations can be found in *NHS Estates Health Building Note No. 46* (DoH 1991).

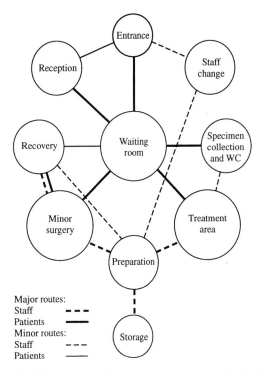

Fig. 1.1. Minor surgery/treatment area room-relationship diagram.

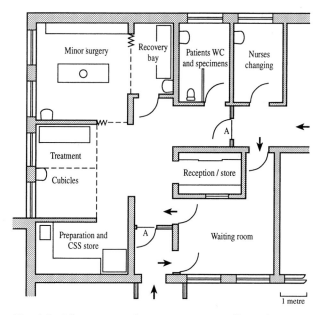

Fig. 1.2. Minor surgery/treatment area—a floor plan (East Oxford Health Centre). A—staff only.

Equipment

Basic equipment for minor surgery should comprise

(1) an adequate selection of instruments;
(2) a simple operating table;
(3) effective light source(s) (preferably shadowless);
(4) sterilization facilities;
(5) instrument trolley(s);
(6) waste disposal facilities;
(7) resuscitation equipment.

More specialized items may also be appropriate, for example,

(1) electrocautery unit;
(2) unipolar diathermy apparatus;
(3) cryotherapy equipment.

Surgical instruments and procedure packs

Individual requirements and preferences will dictate appropriate provision of small instruments for minor surgery in general practice. Suffice it to say that the purchase of instruments of the best quality will ultimately justify the initial additional outlay. Appendix A lists a range of firms who will supply catalogues on request and some, especially if minor surgery facilities are being set up *ab initio*, will offer a discount on bulk purchases. In the experience of the author, a limited number of sets of instruments for specific procedures will simplify laying up for minor operations and these procedure packs are listed as a guide.

Procedure Pack 1. General Purpose (incision/suture)

1 dental syringe (see Chapter 3, Figs 3.2 and 3.3
1 knife handle no. 3 (small) (or use single-use instruments)

1 6″ Mayo needle holder
1 5″ forceps (plain)
1 5″ toothed forceps (fine)
1 5″ curved mosquito forceps
1 5″ straight Spencer Wells
1 skin hook (fine)
1 5″ stitch scissors

Single-use, pre-sterilized scalpel blades available for knife handles sizes 3 and 4 are shown in Figs 1.3 and 1.4.

Procedure Pack 2. Curettage (warts, etc.)
1 dental syringe
1 Volkmann spoon curette (double-ended, small/medium)
1 5″ toothed forceps (fine)
1 5″ straight Mayo scissors

Procedure Pack 3. Ingrowing Toenails
2 Black's files
1 Thwaites' nail nippers
1 Fickling's elevator
1 Beaver handle for chisel blade
1 5″ straight mosquito forceps
6 hardwood applicators with cotton wool wisps

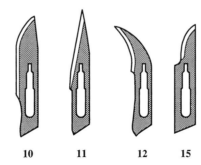

Fig. 1.3. Single-use scalpel blades; handle size no. 3.

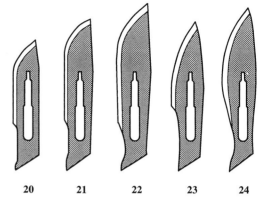

Fig. 1.4. Single-use scalpel blades; handle size no. 4.

1 knife handle no. 3 (small)
1 5″ stitch scissors
1 5″ toothed forceps (fine)
1 5″ dressing forceps

Procedure Pack 4. Meibomian Cyst
2 Tarsal clamps (medium and small)
1 knife handle no. 3 (small)
1 Meibomian curette

Procedure Pack 5. IUCD Insertion
1 Cusco speculum (medium or large)
1 10″ sponge holding forceps
1 10″ single tooth tenaculum
1 uterine sound
2 Hegar dilators (3/4 and 5/6 mm)
1 7″ scissors (blunt/blunt)

Operating Tables

Whilst an ordinary examination couch will often suffice, in the interest of comfort for the patient and convenience of the operator, a simple operating table is preferable, which should, ideally, possess the following features:

(1) there should be an overall tilt facility;
(2) an arm rest and lithotomy stirrups should be available;
(3) it should be mobile but with locking castors;
(4) rising head and drop/removable foot sections;
(5) the height should be adjustable.

Appropriate and relatively inexpensive examples are illustrated in Figs 1.5 and 1.6.

For fixed-height tables, simple mounting steps for patients (Fig. 1.7) are advisable and a further convenience in the minor operations theatre is a small 'kick-about' waste receiver (Fig. 1.8).

Lighting

Heavy, traditional ceiling-mounted operating theatre lights are rarely necessary for general practice surgery and may involve structural

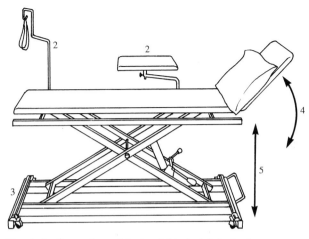

Fig. 1.6. Operating table (variable height). 2. Arm rest and lithotomy stirrups attachment. 3. Locking castors. 4. Adjustable head and foot sections. 5. Height adjustment mechanism.

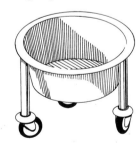

Fig. 1.7. Mounting steps.

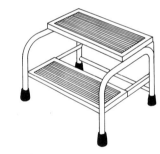

Fig. 1.8. Kick-about receiver.

problems with the reinforcement of ceilings, etc. Simple, wall-mounted or mobile, free-standing lamps of the anglepoise variety are usually adequate for the minor procedures described in this book. Low voltage lamps of the type shown in Fig. 1.9 with quartz halogen bulbs are easily adjustable and ready focused. Two of these, one on either side of the table, ensures a virtually shadow-free field for operating.

Disinfection and sterilization

Traditionally, instruments used in general practice were 'sterilized' by boiling, originally in a kitchen saucepan and latterly in electric hot water boilers. It is now clear that this process will not destroy the spores of some bacteria and the method therefore should only be used for low risk procedures (see Chapter 2). Only steam under pressure or hot air held above critical temperatures for a specified duration will destroy known pathogenic spores, bacteria, and viruses and, thus, achieve satisfactory decontamination of equipment used for higher risk procedures (Hoffman 1987). Table 1.1 shows the recommended temperatures and exposure times for each method. (DoH 1989).

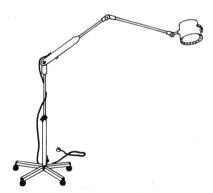

Fig. 1.9. Adjustable halogen spotlight.

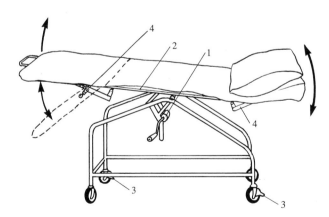

Fig. 1.5. Operating table (fixed height). 1. Table tilt facility. 2. Arm rest and lithotomy stirrups attachment. 3. Locking castors. 4. Adjustable head and foot sections.

Table 1.1. Recommended sterilization times and temperatures for autoclaves and hot air ovens (Morgan 1989, Appendix 3)

	Temperature (°C)	Time (min)
Autoclave	121	15
	126	10
	134	3
Dry heat	160	60
	170	40
	180	20

Steam sterilizers (Autoclaves)

British Standard 3970 (Part 4) (British Standards Institution 1990) lays down the 'specifications for portable steam sterilizers for unwrapped instruments and utensils' and a variety of models are available on the market for use in general practice. In 1988 (revised 1990), the Department of Health (DoH 1990) undertook an evaluation of steam sterilizers and found that the then available appliances fell into three broad groups:

(1) those without preset automatic cycles;
(2) those without the recommended level of instrumentation and cycle monitoring;
(3) those with acceptable performance and basic instrumentation.

Only those models in the third category (inevitably the most expensive) were considered to combine the required instrumentation and performance. Table 1.2 summarizes the findings of the survey in tabular form.

Figure 1.10 illustrates a popular worktop sterilizer that fulfils the requirements for appliances in the third category. It has four available programs:

(1) 134°C without drying;
(2) 121°C without drying;
(3) 134°C with drying;
(4) 121°C with drying.

With drying, two cycles in an hour are possible, whereas without drying four cycles are possible. A further advantage claimed for this model is that, using the 134°C drying program, instruments can be processed in sterilization pouches (View-Packs) although a special rack (Fig. 1.11) must be used. Nevertheless, Department of Health authorities hold reservations (DoH 1989) regarding the effective processing of wrapped loads in worktop steam sterilizers.

Other features of this particular model are electronic program selection, audible and visible cycle completion and malfunction signals, pressure door lock (prevents opening when steam is under pressure), door interlock (program will not commence if door is not secure), pressure and temperature displays, and overheating cut-out.

Hot air sterilization

Figure 1.12 illustrates a contemporary hot air oven. It is available in two sizes and with either manually or electronically controlled programs and air circulation is fan-assisted to avoid hot spots. The capital cost of hot air sterilizers is considerably lower than that of autoclaves but there are a number of disadvantages (see Chapter 2). Satisfactory performance should be monitored by the use of Browne's tubes.

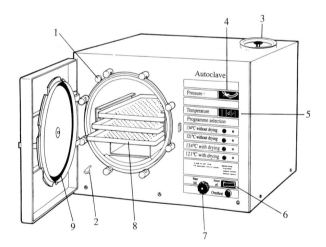

1 Pressure door lock	6 Power switch
2 Door interlock	7 Water fill valve
3 Water reservoir filling point	8 Stainless steel trays
4 Analogue pressure gauge	9 Door seal
5 Display	10 Pouch rack (Fig. 1.11)

Fig. 1.10. A popular steam sterilizer.

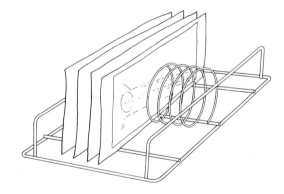

Sterilizing instruments or other metal items in sterilization pouches/bags should only be undertaken using the special pouch rack available as an optional extra (part number 525192). Following washing or ultrasonic cleaning, a suitable number of instruments should be placed in each pouch and the sealed pouches loaded horizontally between the coils of the rack, with no more than one pouch between each coil. When autoclaving Handpieces, they should be placed in an upright position to ensure sterility. Pouches can only be sterilized using the '134°C with drying' cycle, at the end of which the pouches should be dry and may be stored for use at a later date.

Fig. 1.11. Rack for instrument pouches.

Table 1.2. Summary of results of small sterilizer evaluation

Features of sterilizer	Sterilizer model											
	Aesculap 340 ST	Aesculap 354	Benchtop 25	Benchtop 50	Instaclave 25/35	MDT Castle GLS-10	Melag 15ST	Pelton & Crane Validator 8	Prestige 2083	Series 100 '305'	SES LS3	SES 2000
1. Price range	C	E	C	E	E	I	E	F	B	E	F	E
2. Preset automatic cycle	□	□	■	■	■	□	□	■	■	■	■	■
3. User instructions	■	■	■	■	■	■	■	■	■	■	■	■
4. Country of manufacture	FRG	FRG	UK	UK	UK	USA	FRG	USA	UK	UK	UK	UK
5. Sterilizer vessel	▲	▲	▲	■	▲	▲	▲	▲	▲	▲	■	■
6. Safety interlocks	□	□	▲	■	■	□	□	□	▲	■	■	▲
7. Thermocouple entry	□	■	■	■	■	□	□	□	■	■	■	■
8. Chamber furniture and accessories	□	▲	▲	▲	▲	▲	▲	▲	▲	▲	■	■
9. Sterilizer instrumentation	■	■	■	■	■	▲	□	▲	■	■	■	■
10. Control and monitoring	□	□	■	■	▲	▲	□	▲	▲	▲	■	▲
11. Cycle stage/fault indication	□	□	■	■	■	▲	□	▲	■	■	■	■
12. Cycle counter	□	□	□	■	■	□	□	□	□	■	■	□
13. Empty chamber performance	■	▲	□	■	■	■	□	□	■	■	■	■
14. Full load performance	■	■	□	■	■	■	■	□	■	■	■	■
15. Water reservoir temperature	N/A	□	N/A	■	■	▲	N/T	□	N/A	■	▲	▲
16. Chamber water temperature	N/A	N/A	N/T	N/A	■	N/A	N/T	N/A	■	N/A	N/A	N/A
17. Safety cut-outs	□	■	□	■	■	■	▲	■	■	■	■	■
18. Cycle interruption	□	□	▲	■	■	▲	□	□	▲	■	■	▲
19. Surface temperatures	■	■	■	■	■	■	□	■	■	■	■	■
20. Electrical safety	N/I	N/I	▲	▲	▲	N/I	N/I	▲	▲	▲	■	■

Key:
■, meets recommendations.
▲, see report for minor variations from recommendations.
□, does not meet recommendations.

N/A, not applicable.
N/T, not tested—see full report for rationale for not testing.
N/I, no information.

UK, United Kingdom.
G, Germany.
USA, United States of America.

Price bands: A, £0–£300; B, £300–£600; C, £600–£900; D, £900–£1200; E, £1200–£1500; F, £1500–£1800; G, £1800–£2100; H, £2100–£3000; I, £3000+.

Instrument trolleys

Instrument/dressing trolleys are available in a variety of sizes and materials. Of standard height (850 mm, 34″) and depth (450 mm, 18″) they are commonly available as 450 mm (18″), 600 mm (24″), and 750 mm (30″) models. Frames are of tubular steel with castors fitted to the legs. Shelves may be of glass, melamine-faced chipboard, or stainless steel. Although the latter are most expensive, they are the most durable and easily cleaned and flanged

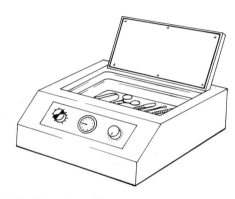

Fig. 1.12. Hot air sterilizer.

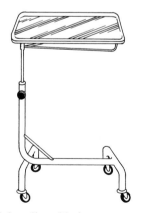

Fig. 1.13. Height-adjustable instrument tray strand.

steel shelves with open corners can double as dressing trays. Drawers in instrument trolleys should be avoided as potential dust traps. A convenient, height-adjustable, mobile instrument tray stand is shown in Fig. 1.13.

Waste disposal facilities

Appropriate arrangements for the collection, storage, and disposal of clinical waste from medical centres is another requirement for approval of premises for reimbursement of rent and rates (*Statement of fees and allowances*, Paragraph 51.13 (NHS General Medical Services 1990)). Although it is the responsibility of general practitioners to ensure the safe disposal of clinical waste, many Family Health Service Authorities (FHSAs) now make their own arrangements for the collection and safe disposal of waste from general practice premises.

Clinical waste, excluding 'sharps', should be

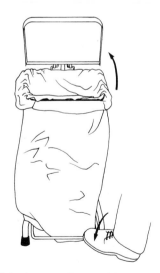

Fig. 1.14. Clinical waste disposal bin.

collected in yellow plastic bags supplied for the purpose in accordance with the Health and Safety Commission colour-coded segregation system, clearly marked 'clinical waste for incineration'. Bags should be mounted in bag bins (Fig. 1.14) the lids for which must be pedal operated. When three-quarters filled, bags should be sealed with plastic adhesive tape and stored in safe conditions whilst awaiting collection for incineration which should normally be arranged at not less than weekly intervals.

Disposal of 'sharps'

Needles, blades and syringes (designed for single-use purposes), broken glass, used glass ampoules, etc., must be placed for disposal in robust, suitably labelled, impenetrable containers again usually supplied by FHSAs in England and Wales. These must not be overfilled and should be securely sealed prior to collection for incineration.

Resuscitation equipment

Zoltie and Hoult (1991), in a survey of 111 practices in a large urban district in the Midlands, found that lack of adequate resuscitation equipment was the second most common reason for failure of premises to reach the minimum standard for approval for minor surgical procedures. Even though inhalational anaesthesia will not be employed in most general practice settings, patients, whether undergoing surgery or not, may occasionally experience vasovagal, epileptiform or anaphylactic reactions on site and appropriate skills and equipment must be on hand to treat such emergencies. Doctors and nurses should attend regular refresher sessions on basic resuscitation techniques and the necessary equipment, regularly checked and tested, should be available. An appropriate list, dependent on the experience and skills of personnel in attendance, might include

(1) Brook airways (three sizes);
(2) assisted breathing bags (for example, Ambu, Weinmann, Vitalograph);
(3) face masks (three sizes);
(4) Guedel airways (three sizes);
(5) oxygen cylinder with regulator valve;
(6) aspirator (hand powered, for example, Vitalograph);
(7) aspiration catheters (various sizes);
(8) laryngoscope (adult and infant blades);
(9) endotracheal tubes (adult and infant sizes);
(10) defibrillator.

Resuscitation equipment outfits of varying complexity are available from medical equipment suppliers. An example is shown in Fig. 1.15 and, in this form, has the advantage that it can be carried by doctors on call out of hours.

In addition, to treat unexpected reactions of varying aetiology, a selection of sterile syringes, needles, and i.v. 'butterfly' needles should be immediately to hand together with

(1) adrenalin 1:1000 solution (1 mg/ml), 1 ml ampoules;
(2) atropine sulphate 600 µg/ml, 1 ml ampoules;
(3) diazepam 5 mg/ml, 2 ml ampoules;
(4) hydrocortisone sodium succinate 100 mg vial, 2 ml sterile water for reconstitution.

It is most important, as items of this nature will only rarely be used, that expiry dates are regularly checked and stocks replenished when necessary.

Specialized equipment
Electrocautery apparatus
Low voltage transformers powering hot wire burners have been used for superficial tissue destruction for many years (Cracknell and Mead 1991). They are simple, inexpensive, and reliable and many (Fig. 1.16) will additionally operate a low voltage light source for endoscopic instruments such as vaginal specula or proctoscopes. Burners are available in a variety of shapes and sizes and are mounted on a switched Mark Hovell handle (Fig. 1.17). Useful only for very superficial tissue destruction procedures and in view of the somewhat offensive smells generated by their use, they have been largely superseded by the type of electrodiathermy apparatus described next.

Electrodiathermy apparatus
Equipment generating electrical current wave-forms suitable for use in surgery has been available for almost a century. Initially, these machines required an indifferent (ground) electrode attached to the patient to complete the effective circuit but, for over 50 years, a development has been available that does not need this sometimes hazardous and inconvenient requisite and which can be used in monoterminal mode. A well-known example of this type of equipment is the Birtcher Hyfrecator (Fig. 1.18). Compact and easily portable, it can be used in a variety of modes (Fig. 1.19) and has a great

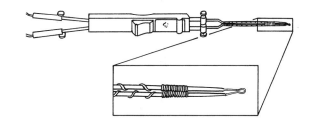
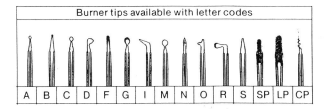

Fig. 1.17. Mark Hovell handles and assorted burner tips.

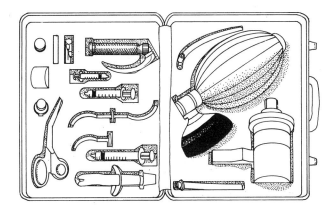

Fig. 1.15. Portable resuscitation kit.

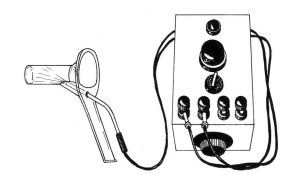

Fig. 1.16. Electrocautery/light transformer.

number of minor surgical applications (see Chapter 7). Various models of this machine are available with a variety of electrodes which are disposable or able to be resterilized. Control can be effected either by a foot switch or a switched handle although the former is necessary for bipolar applications. There are high- and low-power ranges and fully variable current intensity controls. This machine is not, however, designed for 'cutting' diathermy.

The basic electrosurgical techniques available are as follows.

1. 'Desiccation' which involves inserting the tip of the needle electrode into the substance of the lesion before releasing the high frequency discharge. The effect is tissue destruction due to dehydration by evaporating the intracellular fluid. Excessive heat is not generated (unless too high a power setting is used) so surrounding structures are not compromised.

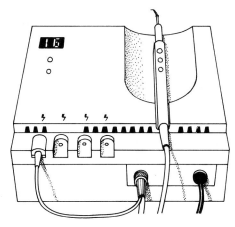

Fig. 1.18. Birtcher Hyfrecator 'Plus' (Model No. 7–797-A).

(a) Monoterminal

The vast majority of HYFRECATOR PLUS procedures use monoterminal techniques. They are easily set up, provide excellent results and do not require any accessory equipment. The current flows from either the High or Low output terminals to the electrode, then passes to the patient. The electricity 'completes the circuit' by seeking its own ground through the patient to the table and across the floor, returning to your unit via the electrical outlet. Monoterminal procedures produce desiccation and fulguration.

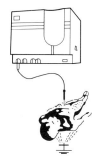

(b) Monopolar

Monopolar applications are less common than monoterminal. Here, the high- frequency current starts from either of the BIPOLAR terminals, then travels through an electrode to your patient, where it exits through a Dispersive Patient Plate and returns directly to the unit via the other BIPOLAR terminal. Monopolar applications produce coagulation.

NOTE: The terms 'Monoterminal' and 'Monopolar' are frequently interchanged. Both should really be called 'Monoterminal'. The HYFRECATOR PLUS uses AC current which constantly changes its direction of flow. Technically there are no 'poles'.

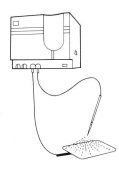

(c) Bipolar

For Bipolar configurations, the current flow is similar to monoterminal techniques, except the electricity never spreads deeply into the tissue. Instead, forceps — or other highly specialized electrodes — keep the current flow on the surface, travelling from one tine of the forceps to the other. Bipolar techniques produce *coagulation*.

NOTE: Bipolar forcep procedures require the use of a Footswitch.

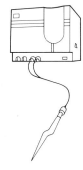

Fig. 1.19. Hyfrecator 'Plus' function modes. (a) Monoterminal configuration, (b) monopolar configuration, (c) bipolar configuration.

2. 'Fulgaration' is achieved by holding the tip of the electrode a short distance from the lesion so that the required effect is attained by an electric spark (arc) between the needle and the skin surface. Tissue destruction is thus limited to a shallow area under the electrode and the formation of a thin eschar.

3. 'Coagulation' which is useful for the control of superficial haemorrhage, is best achieved using a ball electrode, rather than a needle, held in close proximity to an oozing surface. Bleeding from identified blood vessels can be controlled more effectively by means of bipolar coagulation using insulated forceps obtainable from the suppliers.

As with the use of most specialized equipment, there is a learning curve towards the realization of the full potential of electrosurgical techniques. The beginner should experiment initially, perhaps, on something like a pig's ear or trotter (obtainable from most family butchers at nominal expense) before progressing to human subjects.

Cryosurgery equipment

Cryotherapy (freezing) is an alternative method for the treatment of many superficial, benign dermatological lesions seen in general practice (Hopkins 1983; Cracknell and Mead 1991). It is a simple procedure that needs neither aseptic precautions nor the prior injection of local anaesthetic. Tissue destruction is achieved by rapid cooling causing the formation of intracellular ice crystals, followed by slow thawing which results in subsequent necrosis. Freezing may be accomplished reliably by the rapid expansion of gases such as carbon dioxide, nitrous oxide, or nitrogen held either in the compressed or the liquid state. The rapid evaporation of organic liquids such as ethyl chloride or dimethyl ether will also produce low temperatures but, since a temperature of −30°C is required to achieve reliable tissue destruction, the application of a gas in liquid form is most commonly used to ensure satisfactory results, for example, nitrogen (boiling point −196°C) or nitrous oxide (−85°C).

Nitrous oxide, being only available in high pressure cylinders, requires relatively expensive cryoprobe apparatus for its use but liquid nitrogen, being completely inert and readily available in liquid form, offers a simple, inexpensive, effective, and safe medium for local application. The liquid gas is readily available from commercial sources but can often be obtained at a nominal charge locally from a district hospital. Whilst it can be transported in a

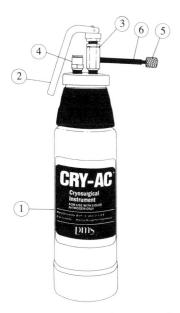

Fig. 1.20. Liquid nitrogen cryotherapy equipment. 1. Vacuum insulated flask. 2. Trigger lever. 3. Control valve. 4. Pressure relief valve. 5. Spray tip. 6. Discharge tube.

domestic thermos flask, it is more sensible to invest in a vented steel transport vessel to avoid accidental loss, spillages, and possible injury. Liquid nitrogen can be simply applied (see the illustrated procedure 'cryotherapy of warts, moles, and keratoses', in Chapter 7, pp. 102, 103) with a cotton wool bud or by using more sophisticated cryotherapy equipment (Fig. 1.20). Since transport vessels are vented, the liquid gas will slowly disperse; as an approximate guide, a vessel holding 500 ml liquid nitrogen will be exhausted within 24 h so the treatment of suitable conditions is best planned on a sessional basis.

When using destructive cryotherapy techniques, adequate exposure times must be learnt by experience and it is sensible to err on the side of underexposure until judgement has developed. In this way damage to deeper structures such as blood vessels, nerves, and tendons is avoided. If destruction of the lesion is not achieved initially, the patient should return again for treatments of increasing duration. Always wear gloves when handling liquid nitrogen to avoid self-injury and note that some cryotherapy guns will not function effectively if tilted more than 45° from the vertical axis.

References

British Standards Institution (1990). *Transportable steam sterilisers for unwrapped instruments and utensils*. British Standard 3970 (Part 4), B.S.I., Milton Keynes.

Cracknell, I. and Mead, M. (1991). Electrocautery and cryocautery. *Update*, **42**, 1181–4.

Department of Health (1989). *Safety Action Bulletin No. 52. 'Instrument and utensil' steam sterilisers: misuse*. DoH, London.

Department of Health (1990). *Health Equipment Information Publication No. 196. An evaluation of portable steam sterilisers for unwrapped instruments and utensils*. HMSO, London.

Department of Health (1991). *National Health Service Estates: Health Building Note No. 46*. HMSO, London.

Hoffman, P. N. (1987). Decontamination of equipment in general practice. *Practitioner*, **231**, 1411–15.

Hopkins, P. (1983). Cryosurgery by the general practitioner. *Practitioner*, **227**, 1861–73.

Morgan, D. (ed.) (1989). *A code of practice for sterilisation of instruments and control of cross infection*. British Medical Association, London.

National Health Service General Medical Services (1990). *Statement of fees and allowances payable to general medical practitioners in England and Wales from 1 April 1990*. Department of Health Welsh Office, London.

Zoltie, N. and Hoult, G. (1991). Adequacy of general practitioners' premises for minor surgery. *British Medical Journal*, **302**, 941–2.

Further reading

Cammock, R. (1973). *Health centres—reception, waiting and patient call*. HMSO, London.

Cammock, R. (1981). *Primary health care buildings*. Architectural Press, London.

Cammock, R. and Grayson, H. (1979). *Utilisation of treatment suites in health centres and group practice*. Medical Architecture Research Unit, North London Polytechnic, London.

Department of Health (1987). *Draft building note: general medical practice premises for the provision of primary health care services*. DoH, London.

National Building Agency/College of General Practitioners (1970). *Design guide for medical group practice centres*. NBA/RCGP, London.

Scottish Home and Health Department (1973). *Design guide: health centres in Scotland*. HMSO, Edinburgh.

Snook, R. (1985). Minor surgery in general practice: are you equipped for the job? *MIMS Magazine*, 15 December, 15–19.

Appendix A: suppliers of medical equipment and instruments

Instruments and general equipment
Ash Instruments Division, Dentsply Ltd, 9, Madlease Estate, Bristol Road, Gloucester GL1 5SG.

John Bell & Croyden, 52–54, Wigmore Street, London W1H 0AU. Tel: 071 935 555.

Bridge Medical Direct, 118, Chatham Street, Reading, Berkshire RG1 7HT. Tel: 0734 393433.

'Doctor' Buylines, Reed Business Publishing Group, Quadrant House, The Quadrant, Sutton, Surrey SM2 5AS.

Downs Surgical Plc., Church Path, Mitcham, Surrey CR4 3UE. Tel: 081 648 6291.

Eschmann Bros & Walsh Ltd, Equipment Division, Peter Road, Lancing, West Sussex BN15 8TJ. Tel: 0903 753322.

Gallops Trolleys, Rock-a-Nore Road, Hastings, East Sussex TN34 3DW. Tel: 0424 421485.

Philip Harris Medical, Hazelwell Lane, Stirchley, Birmingham B30 2PS. Tel: 021 433 3030.

Holborn Surgical Instrument Co. Dolphin Works, Margate Road, Broadstairs, Kent CT10 2QQ. Tel: 0843 61418.

Macarthy's Surgical, Selinas Lane, Dagenham, Essex RM8 1QD. Tel: 081 593 7511.

Porter Nash Medical, 116, Wigmore Street, London W1H 9FD. Tel: 071 487 4288.

Reed Healthcare Communications Ltd, Buylines, 13–21, High Street, Guildford, Surrey GU1 3DX.

Rocket of London, Imperial Way, Watford, Hertfordshire WD2 4XX. Tel: 0923 39791.

Seward Medical Ltd, UAC House, Blackfriars Road, London SE1 9UG. Tel: 071 928 9431.

Charles, F. Thackray Ltd, (Thackraycare Products), 45–47, Great George Street, Leeds LS1 3BB. Tel: 0532 788145.

Williams Medical Supplies, Unit H6, Springhead Enterprise Park, Springhead Road, Northfleet, Gravesend, Kent DA11 8HD. Tel: 0474 535330.

Cautery and diathermy
Rimmer Bros. Ltd, 18–19, Aylesbury Street, Clerkenwell, London EC1R 2OD. Tel: 071 251 6494.

Schuco International London Ltd, Lyndhurst Avenue, Woodhouse Road, London N12 0NE. Tel: 081 368 1642.

Cryosurgery equipment
Cryogenic Technology Ltd, Unit 2, Goods Road, Belper, Derbyshire DE5 1UU. Tel: 0773 821515.

Galderma (UK) Ltd, Imperial Way, Hertfordshire WD2 4YR. Tel: 0923 210180.

Healthcare Advisory Services, Holmsdale, Tokers Green Lane, Kidmore End, Reading RG4 9EB. Tel: 0734 722696.

Practice Management Systems Ltd, 145b, Hughenden Road, High Wycombe, Buckinghamshire HP13 5PN. Tel: 0494 474811.

Miscellaneous
Chiropody and podiatry
Mediforce, Carr House, Carrbottom Road, Bradford BD5 9BJ. Tel: 0274 732328.

Biopsy punches
Steifel Laboratories (UK) Ltd, Holtspur Lane, Woodburn Green, High Wycombe, Buckinghamshire HP10 0AU. Tel: 06285 24966.

Minor surgery simulator kits
Limbs & Things Ltd, Radnor Business Centre, Radnor Road, Horfield, Bristol BS7 8QS. Tel: 0272 446466.

Biohazard Spill Kits
Guest Medical Ltd., Enterprize Way, Edenbridge, Kent TN8 6EW. Tel: 0732 867466.

2 Control of infection

Disinfection and sterilization

A basic principle of medicine through the ages has been that of *non nocere* (do no harm), a concept which must include the risk of the introduction of infection in the course of any invasive procedure. Whilst bacterial vectors have been recognized and countered for over a century, the recent advent of potentially lethal viral infections such as HIV and hepatitis B have been accompanied by the realization that reciprocal transmission may now prove a hazard to surgeons and assistants (including nurses) as well as to patients (DHSS 1987).

In the preparation of equipment and instruments for minor operations in general practice, it is important to distinguish (Hoffman 1987) between sterilization (total freedom from microbes and spores) and disinfection (the eradication of microbes, but not necessarily spores) and to relate the method of decontamination to the risk category of the procedure proposed (Hoffman *et al.* 1988). The same authors, in a survey of 20 general practices in four different areas of England, found that in only just over half (56 per cent) of the decontamination procedures investigated could the results be considered completely satisfactory. They made recommendations (Table 2.1) relating procedure risk to decontamination method which should form appropriate guidelines for practitioners undertaking minor surgery on their practice premises.

Available methods for decontamination of instruments and equipment will now be briefly summarized (see also Hoffman 1987; Morgan 1989).

Table 2.1. Recommended methods for instrument decontamination and usage in general practice (Hoffman *et al.* 1988)

	Recommended methods	Acceptable alternatives
High risk items Surgical scissors and forceps Stitch cutters Intra-uterine device sets Uterine sounds Tenacula Neurological examination pins	Sterilize or single use (pre-sterile)	None
Medium risk items Vaginal specula Fitting rings/diaphragms Ring pessaries Proctoscopes/sigmoidoscopes Auriscope 'nozzles' Laryngeal mirrors Nasal specula Tongue depressors Peak flow meter mouthpieces	Sterilize or single use	Boil if suitable or none
Thermometers—oral-rectal	Seventy per cent alcohol for for 10 min or single use	None
Low risk items Ear syringe nozzles	Sterilize or boil	Chemical disinfection or wash
Skin thermometers	Seventy per cent alcohol for 10 min or single use	Wash

Hospital-based central sterile supply service (CSSD)

This type of service is the ideal (Sims 1985) if it can be negotiated with a local hospital. It is likely to be expensive however, since multiple procedure packs of various types (see Chapter 1) will be required and charges for capital expenditure on instruments as well as for processing will be incurred. Problems may also be experienced relating to transport and facilities will be required for holding both used and unused equipment. An added advantage, however, is that sterile cotton drapes and dressing towels can also be processed.

Worktop autoclaves (steam sterilization under pressure)

Although initially expensive, modern worktop steam sterilizers are safe and reliable. The availability and characteristics of various models have been discussed in Chapter 1. If the use of sealed instrument packs, for example, View-Pack (Smith Brothers (Whitehaven) Ltd), is contemplated, the autoclave must have an operating temperature of 134 °C with a drying cycle and must be equipped with a special rack for the envelopes (Fig. 1.11).[†] If envelopes are not employed, instruments should be used immediately after cooling or, if laid out on trays and covered by sterile sheets, within 3 h. Cotton towels cannot be sterilized effectively in worktop autoclaves. Steam sterilizers must be inspected under a maintenance contract at regular intervals and their performance parameters checked. It is also important to remember that disinfection of instruments will not be satisfactory unless they are properly cleaned (see below) prior to processing.

Hot air ovens

Since heat transference is far more efficient by steam than by dry heat, hot air ovens need higher operating temperatures and longer cycles than autoclaves. Sixty minutes holding time at 160 °C or 20 min at 180 °C is required and holding times must commence only when the operating temperature has been reached. Although of lower initial cost compared with autoclaves, in view of the higher temperatures required, cooling times for instruments may often be inconveniently prolonged. Procedure packs can be fashioned from aluminium kitchen foil but cotton or paper goods should not be

---

[†] But see DOH (1989). *Safety action bulletin no. 52. 'Instrument and utensil' steam/sterilisers: misuse.* DoH, London.

included because of the risk of charring. A domestic oven can, in exceptional circumstances, be used for hot air sterilization of instruments but a Brown's tube must always be included which, by colour change, will confirm that the decontamination process has been effective.

Hot water disinfectors

Hot water boilers (often euphemistically called 'sterilizers') cannot achieve the decontamination necessary for high risk procedure since they cannot guarantee the destruction of bacterial spores. Owing to rapid heat transference, instruments can, however, be effectively disinfected by immersion for 5 min in visibly boiling water. Most boilers are fitted with a perforated draining tray on which instruments can cool after removal from the boiler. Distilled, pre-boiled, or de-ionized water should be used to prevent furring of the instruments by lime scale.

Chemical disinfection

Chemical disinfection is the least reliable of the available methods but must sometimes be used for equipment that would be damaged or destroyed by heat. Hypochlorite solutions, useful for the disinfection of working surfaces (see below), is corrosive to metals and quickly discolours even stainless steel instruments. Glutaraldehyde or formaldehyde both possess highly irritant vapours and must only be used in carefully controlled circumstances (Aw and Barnes 1990). Alcohols, in the form of industrial methylated spirit (70 per cent ethanol plus 5 per cent wood naphtha) or isopropanol (70 per cent isopropyl alcohol) are effective disinfectants and 10 min immersion of instruments is sufficient. An advantage is that no cooling-off period is necessary but residual alcohol should be rinsed away using sterile water or saline, a

particularly important precaution if cautery or diathermy is to be used since alcohols are highly inflammable! Moreover, they do not penetrate well into organic matter so efficient pre-cleaning of equipment is mandatory.

Disposable (single-use) instruments

An increasing range of single-use instruments, pre-sterilized by gamma radiation, is now available. Disposable gloves and standard size syringes and needles have long been available from FHSAs and, more recently, disposable vaginal specula and proctoscopes. A range of suture materials (Chapter 5, Appendix B) and dressing packs (Chapter 5, Appendix C) are available on prescription and costs can be reclaimed under NHS General Medical Services (1990) arrangements (*Statement of fees and allowances*, Paragraph 44.1 (a)). The more elaborate dressing packs contain plastic gallipots and several pairs of disposable dressing forceps. Disposable scalpels, stitch scissors, biopsy punches, etc., are also available but the convenience of these has to be set against the costs, which may not be reclaimable.

Preparation for minor surgery

Since minor surgical procedures in general practice will not involve penetration of body cavities, conventional hospital operating theatre precautions and sterile environments are not necessary. The following points may, however, be relevant.

Personal protection

GP surgeons should ensure that they have been actively immunized against poliomyelitis, tetanus, and hepatitis B and that seroconversion to the latter has been achieved. Reinforcing doses should be accepted when due.

Gowns

Sterile gowns are unnecessary but the surgeon should wear a disposable plastic apron to prevent contamination and splashing of his clothing which might be stained, for example, when using an iodine-based surgical scrub or skin cleanser.

Masks

Masks for general practitioner surgeons and nurses are not now considered necessary when performing simple external procedures (Orr 1981).

Hand washing

Taylor (1978) has shown that conventional hand washing often misses important areas, especially the fingertips and thumbs, but Ayliffe *et al.* (1978) have recommended a routine that is simple, quick, and effective (Fig. 2.1). This sequence should be repeated three times under running water using an antiseptic surfactant solution containing chlorhexidine (Hibiscrub) or povidone–iodine (Betadine), then rinsing thoroughly and drying on sterile paper towels. If the application of an alcoholic solution (Hibisol, Betadine alcoholic solution) is used instead of an aqueous surfactant, continue the same routine repeatedly until the liquid has evaporated and the skin is dry.

The wash routine should be performed as follows.

1. Add an appropriate quantity of the favoured surfactant solution to the palmar surface of one hand and rub and hands together.
2. Interlace the fingers whilst rubbing, right palmar surface over left dorsal. (Repeat with left palmar surface over right dorsal.)
3. Interlace fingers palm to palm whilst rubbing.
4. Work knuckles of left hand into right palm then knuckles of right hand into left palm.

5. Rub right thumb with palm and fingers on left hand. (Repeat with left thumb and right palm.)
6. Work right hand fingertips into left palm. (Repeat with left hand fingertips into right palm.)

Gloves

Sterile rubber or polyvinyl surgical gloves should always be worn by the surgeon if the procedure proposed involves actual or potential contact with

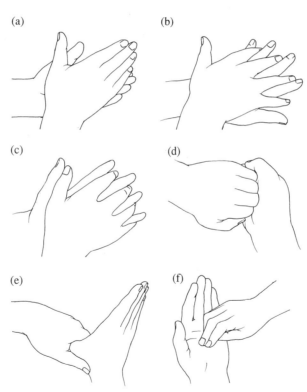

(a) (b) (c) (d) (e) (f)

Fig. 2.1. A simple, effective scrub-up routine (after Ayliffe *et al.* 1978).

body fluids such as blood, urine, saliva, faeces, or semen, both for the protection of the operator and as part of routine aseptic technique. Richmond *et al.* (1992) have drawn attention to the high incidence of accidental needle perforations of gloves occurring in the course of minor surgery so, when operating on patients known or suspected of being hepatitis B carriers or HIV positive, two pairs of sterile gloves should be worn, a precaution which will substantially reduce the risk of needle stick injuries (Doyle *et al.* 1992). However, if in spite of such provisions, a needle stick injury should occur, the procedures laid down by the Expert Advisory Group on AIDS (UK Health Departments 1990) should be followed implicitly. When cleaning instruments and equipment after use or dealing with spillages (see below) stout domestic rubber gloves should be worn for additional protection.

Skin preparation for operation

This subject has been comprehensively reviewed by Lowbury (1973) and Ayliffe (1980). Adequate inhibition of bacterial activity can be achieved within 30 s by the application of 70 per cent ethyl or isopropyl alcohol. It is more usual, however, to use alcohol-based preparations containing an added antibacterial agent such as chlorhexidine 0.5 per cent (Hibisol) or povidone-iodine 10 per cent (Betadine). The latter has the added advantage, by virtue of its colour, of indicating the area that has been prepared and these alcohol-based agents will provide effective antibacterial activity on the skin for several hours (Lilly *et al.* 1979). There is some evidence (Niedner and Schöpf 1986) that some antiseptics particularly chlorhexidine, have an inhibitory effect on wound healing and, thus, should not be used for sluicing out wounds with the object of reducing secondary infection. Evans (1992) has reported a rare case of anaphylaxis following the topical application of chlorhexidine. Furthermore, alcoholic cleansing solutions should *not* be used when the use of electrocautery or diathermy is anticipated for fear of ignition. Indeed, when such appliances are used for the treatment of superficial lesions such as warts, papillomata, naevi, etc., additional skin sterilization is not normally necessary.

When surgery involving mucous membranes (for example, mouth, eye, vagina, anus) is contemplated, water-based antiseptic solutions should be used which have, in addition, a detergent action. Cetrimide 15 per cent with chlorhexidine gluconate 1.5 per cent (Savlon Hospital Concentrate) diluted 1:30 with sterile water is appropriate for this purpose and is available ready diluted in sterile 25 and 100 ml sachets (Savlodil, Savloclens).

Surgical Drapes

Cotton operating sheets with a central aperture are best but rarely available in general practice unless there is access to the hospital-based central sterile supply service. Even if available, they cannot be resterilized adequately in worktop autoclaves and hot air ovens quickly destroy them. However, standard sterile dressing packs always contain a paper towel from which a makeshift sheet can be fashioned as follows.

(1) When scrubbed up, open out the paper towel taken from the dressing pack.
(2) Fold twice as shown in Fig. 2.2 and cut off the corner with sterile scissors.
(3) Open out the sheet again and lay the fenestration over the operation site as required.

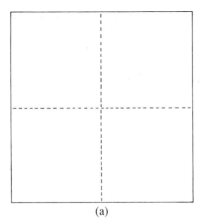

(a)

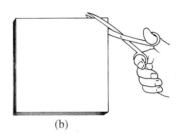

(b)

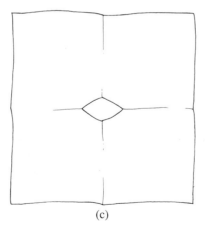

(c)

Fig. 2.2. A makeshift operation sheet.

Cleaning and storage of instruments

After use, all instruments must be freed from organic matter prior to reuse or storage. This can be achieved by the use of an ultrasonic cleaning bath (Brown 1988), or more economically, if less efficiently, by thorough washing in warm water with added household detergent. For the latter option, the operative should wear stout domestic rubber gloves and the process should be undertaken in a sink not used for other purposes. Removal of waste products is facilitated by the use of a synthetic bristle brush or a brass wire brush such as is often used for refurbishing suede footwear. After washing, rinse equipment thoroughly under running hot water and dry off with absorbent kitchen paper. Items may then be stored for future use or packed in View-Pack envelopes prior to resterilization.

Work surfaces

After use, work surfaces such as worktops, trolleys, and instrument trays should be decontaminated using either 70 per cent alcohol or hypochlorite solution (1000 parts per million (p.p.m.) available chlorine (avCl). Leave the reagent in contact with the surface for 3 min, then rinse off and dry with absorbent paper. If body fluids such as blood or pus are visible, use fresh hypochlorite solution (10 000 p.p.m. avCl) for 10 min and dispose of the cloth for incineration afterwards. When using hypochlorite solutions always wear stout domestic rubber gloves to avoid skin maceration.

Dealing with spillages

Gross spillages of body fluids should be contained by using hypochlorite in granular form (sodium dichloroisocyanurate) which can then be swept into a makeshift paper or cardboard receptacle for disposal by incineration. Again, stout household gloves must always be worn and the surface involved treated with hypochlorite solution 10 000 p.p.m. avCl for 10 min as described above. Before decontamination, broken glass (if any) should first be carefully picked out with disposable forceps and placed into a 'sharps' box for safe disposal. Biohazard spillage kits are commercially available (Chapter 1, Appendix A).

References

Aw, T. C. and Barnes, A. (1990). Occupational health and the use of chemical disinfectants: what is needed under COSHH regulations. *Institute of Sterile Services Mangement Journal*, **11**, 7–8.

Ayliffe, G. A. J. (1980). Effect of antibacterial agents on the flora of the skin. *Journal of Hospital Infection*, **11**, 111–24.

Ayliffe, G. A. J., Babb, J. R., and Quoraishi, A. H. A. (1978). A test for 'hygienic' hand disinfection. *Journal of Clinical Pathology*, **31**, 923–8.

Brown, J. S. (1988). An ultrasonic cleaning bath in general practice. *The Practitioner*, **232**, 377.

Department of Health (1987). *Decontamination of equipment, linen or other surfaces contaminated with hepatitis B or HIV virus*. DHSS HN(87)1, London.

Doyle, P. M., Alvi, S., and Johanson, R. (1992). The effectiveness of double-gloving in obstetrics and gynaecology. *British Journal of Obstetrics and Gynaecology*, **99**, 83–4.

Evans, R. J. (1992). Acute anaphylaxis due to topical chlorhexidine acetate. *British Medical Journal*, **304**, 686.

Hoffman, P. N. (1987). Decontamination of equipment in general practice. *Practitioner*, **231**, 1411–15.

Hoffman, P. N., Cooke, E. M., Larkin, D. P., Southgate, L. J. *et al.* (1988). Control of infection in general practice: a survey and recommendations. *British Medical Journal*, **297**, 34–6.

Lilly, H. A., Lowbury, E. J. L., Wilkins, M. D., and Zaggy, A. (1979). Delayed antimicrobial effects of skin disinfection by alcohol. *Journal of Hygiene (Cambridge)*, **82**, 497–500.

Lowbury, E. J. L., (1973). Skin preparation for operation. *British Journal of Hospital Medicine*, **10**, 627–34.

Morgan, D. (ed.) (1989). *A code of practice for sterilisation of instruments and control of cross infection*. British Medical Association, London.

National Health Service General Medical Services (1990). *Statement of fees and allowances payable to general medical practitioners in England and Wales from 1 April, 1990*. Department of Health Welsh Office, London.

Niedner, R. and Schöpf, E. (1986). Inhibition of wound healing by antiseptics. *British Journal of Dermatology*, **115**, 31–41.

Orr, N. W. M. (1981). Is a mask necessary in the operating theatre? *Annals of the Royal College of Surgeons of England*, **63**, 390–2.

Richmond, P. W., McCabe, M., Davies, J. P. and Thomas, D. M. (1992). Perforation of gloves in an accident and emergency department. *British Medical Journal*, **304**, 879–80.

Sims, P. A. (1985). Providing sterilized instrument packs for general practice. *Journal of the Royal College of General Practitioners*, **35**, 298.

Taylor, L. J. (1978). An evaluation of hand-washing techniques. *Nursing Times*, **74**, 54–5, 108–10.

UK Health Departments (1990). *Guidance for clinical health care workers: protection against infection with HIV and hepatitis viruses*. Recommendations of the Expert Advisory Group on AIDS, HMSO, London.

3 Analgesia for minor surgical procedures

Properties of local anaesthetic agents

A major criterion for minor surgical procedures undertaken in general practice is that they should not require the induction of general anaesthesia. It is therefore most important that doctors should have a satisfactory understanding of the principles and characteristics of local anaesthetic preparations and the techniques appropriate to their use.

Local anaesthetic drugs act by causing a reversible inhibition of conduction along nerve fibres. The drugs used vary widely in their potency, toxicity, duration of action, stability, solubility, and ability to penetrate the integument. These variations determine their suitability for use by various methods and routes, for example, by topical application, dermal infiltration, nerve block, intravenous regional anaesthesia, etc. In estimating the safe dosage it is important to take into account the rate at which they are absorbed and excreted as well as their potency and the clinical indication. The patient's age, weight and physique, the vascularity of the area involved, and the required duration of effect are other factors which must be considered.

There are two broad groups of drugs available with local anaesthetic properties, the ester and the amide types. The earliest to be used were the esters which included cocaine, novocaine, and tetracaine. Cocaine was popular in earlier years in view of its topical efficacy and additional vasoconstrictor properties which made it especially useful for oral and nasopharyngeal surgery. The esters have an advantage in that they are metabolized in tissue plasma but, unfortunately, they carry with it an increased risk of the development of allergic reactions, especially when used topically. Nowadays, the amide group (lignocaine, bupivacaine, prilocaine, etc.) is preferred, mainly in view of the low incidence of allergy. They are, however, metabolized in the liver so should be used with extra caution in patients with impaired hepatic function.

Some of the features of local anaesthetics in common use are shown in Table 3.1. Although speed and duration of action are important considerations affecting the selection of an agent for local analgesia, the rate of uptake into the general circulation is the main factor determining toxicity. There is thus a maximum dose for each preparation, dependent on the patient's weight, which should not be exceeded. Lignocaine is the drug of choice for most minor surgical procedures today although bupivacaine has a place where long duration of action and prolonged post-operative analgesia is required, for example, for nerve blocks. Prilocaine is mostly reserved for regional intravenous techniques (for example, Bier's block) on account of its rapid clearance rate. For lignocaine, Kelly and Henderson (1983) have designed a useful nomogram (Fig. 3.1) indicating the maximum volume of the various available dilutions that can be administered according to the patient's weight. The limits are thus relatively high, especially if the lower concentrations are used and these are unlikely to be exceeded for most minor surface procedures.

Toxic effects of amide-type anaesthetics may include warning symptoms such as tinnitus, light-headedness, metallic taste, nausea, vomiting or diplopia. More serious sequelae are nystagmus, dysphasia, muscular fasciculation or epileptiform

Table 3.1. Characteristics, dosage, and availability of local anaesthetic agents

	Lignocaine	Bupivacaine	Prilocaine
Proprietary name	(Xylocaine)	(Marcain)	(Citanest)
Speed of action	Quick	Slow	Average
Duration of effect	Average	Long	Short
Clearance rate	Average	Slow	Fast
Vasodilator effect	Neutral	Increased	Increased
Available solution strengths (%)			
0.25		+	
0.5	+	+	+
0.75		+	
1.0	+		+
2.0	+		+
Recommended maximum dose (mg/kg)	3	2	10
Maximum dose (70 kg adult) in mg			
Without adrenalin	200	140	400
With adrenalin	500	280	600
Indications	Infiltration	Nerve blocks	Regional i.v. use

seizures. The latter are likely only if something in the order of double the safe limit has been exceeded. In either case, infiltration should be discontinued immediately and the patient rested in the recovery position until the symptoms have resolved.

Use of adrenalin

Apart from cocaine, most local anaesthetics produce a degree of vasodilatation which, by increasing the rate of absorption of the drug, reduces the duration of action and may increase the risk of toxic side-effects. The addition of a vasoconstrictor to the solution therefore, by retarding diffusion, will

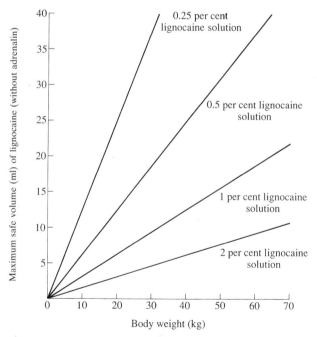

Fig. 3.1. Maximum safe volume of plain lignocaine according to body weight; Kelly and Henderson (1983).

Table 3.2. The advantages and disadvantages of using adrenalin with local anaesthetic agents

Advantages	Disadvantages
Increased duration of analgesia	Risk of adrenergic side-effects
Smaller volume of anaesthetic agent required	Infiltration may be more painful
Reduced haemorrhage at the operation site	Risk of reactionary haemorrhage following the procedure
Reduced risk of toxic effects from anaesthetic reagent	Risk of tissue necrosis in certain areas

counteract these unwanted effects. Smaller quantities of the agent can thus be used and an added benefit may be the reduction of haemorrhage encountered when undertaking superficial procedures, although it is important to watch for reactionary haemorrhage when the vasoconstrictor effect wears off. Adrenalin (epinephrine) 1 : 200 000 (0.5 mg/100 ml) is available as an optional constituent in most proprietary local anaesthetic solutions. Nevertheless, there are some important contraindications to its use, particularly in situations where prolonged vasoconstriction could give rise to ischaemia and subsequent tissue necrosis. For example, adrenalin should **never** be used in local anaesthetic solutions for procedures involving fingers and toes, the nose, the nipple, or the glans penis. It should also be used with caution in patients suffering from or on medication for hypertension and cardiac conditions. The advantages and disadvantages of using adrenalin with local anaesthetic agents are summarized in Table 3.2 but a basic rule of thumb is to use it unless there is a specified contraindication.

In summary, toxic reactions to local anaesthetic solutions can be avoided by:

(1) using the lowest concentration of anaesthetic appropriate to the task;

(2) using the lowest volume of solution necessary;

(3) using adrenalin-containing solutions unless contraindicated;

(4) allowing sufficient time for the solution to take effect;

(5) using nerve blocks wherever possible

Local Anaesthetic Techniques

Topical analgesia

EMLA cream

EMLA cream is a eutectic mixture of lignocaine 2.5 per cent and prilocaine 2.5 per cent which can be useful in situations when the integument is thin, for example, on the lip or near the anus or for the production of superficial analgesia prior to intradermal infiltration in nervous subjects. For best effect, it needs to be applied fairly liberally and under an occlusive dressing for not less than 2 h prior to surgery. For this reason its role is somewhat limited.

Lignocaine

Lignocaine (Xylocaine) 10 per cent aerosol spray is available in a metered dose container (10 mg per dose, 800 doses per container). It is insufficiently penetrative for dermal use but quite rapidly effective on mucosal surfaces such as in the mouth or on the vulva and the anus. Where deeper analgesia is required in these situations, it should be followed by infiltration of a lignocaine solution containing adrenalin.

Refrigerant sprays
Refrigerant sprays such as ethyl chloride, dimethyl ether (Histofreezer), dichlorotetrafluoroethane (Frigiderm), and liquid nitrogen are effective in producing transient surface analgesia which lasts for a few seconds only. This may be of sufficient duration for the incision of a very superficial abscess or haematoma or the insertion of a needle for local infiltration in a very apprehensive patient but rarely for more complex procedures. It should be remembered that ethyl chloride is inflammable and also has general anaesthetic properties if inhaled. It should therefore only be used in well-ventilated premises and for procedures where the use of electrocautery or diathermy is not contemplated. Dichlorotetrafluoroethane is a fluorinated hydrocarbon and, thus, now contraindicated for ecological reasons.

Topical ophthalmic preparations
These include amethocaine, oxybuprocaine (Benoxinate), lignocaine, and proxymetacaine (Ophthaine). These are all available in the 'Minims' (Smith & Nephew) formulation for single-dose use. Proxymetacaine, when instilled into the conjunctival sac, stings less than other preparations so may be more suitable for use in children. Lignocaine (4 per cent) is available containing fluorescein (0.25 per cent) in the Minims series and is thus particularly useful in the differential diagnosis of corneal lesions.

Invasive Local Anaesthetic Techniques
For the purposes of this section, please assume that lignocaine 1 per cent solution with 1 : 200 000 adrenalin is to be used unless otherwise specified. It is available in 2.2 ml syringe cartridges, 5 and 10 ml glass ampoules, and also in 20 ml rubber-capped vials. The latter must not be employed for multi-patient use owing to the risk of cross-infection.

Field blocks

Equipment
For small areas, a dental syringe is most convenient (Figs 3.2 and 3.3). The double-ended, 30 gauge, 30 mm needles are finer, longer, and more easily manipulated than the smallest (25 gauge, 17 mm,

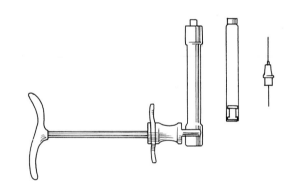

Fig. 3.2. Dental syringe (components).

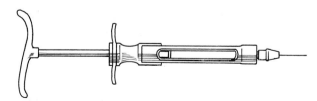

Fig. 3.3. Dental syringe (assembled).

orange mount) needles available to NHS practitioners in the UK. A disadvantage of the dental syringe, however, is that aspiration to check whether a blood vessel has been entered by the needle is not possible. However, the infiltration techniques described below should minimize this risk. For most superficial procedures, two 2.2 ml cartridges of lignocaine 1 per cent with adrenalin will be sufficient to anaesthetize the planned area of operation but, for more extensive activities requiring larger volumes of anaesthetic solution (for example, episiotomy repair), standard 10 or 20 ml sterile plastic disposable syringes with 17 gauge (green mount) or 21 gauge (blue mount) needles should be used.

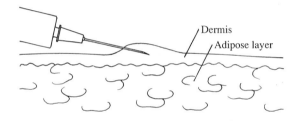

Fig. 3.4. Infiltration technique: intradermal.

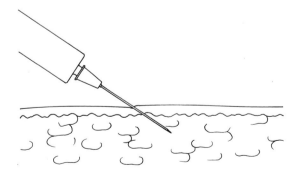

Fig. 3.5. Infiltration technique: subcutaneous.

Technique

For many procedures, local anaesthesia can be established prior to scrubbing up and setting out of instruments. This gives the solution sufficient time to work effectively and reduces waiting time for the operator.

Infiltration of the field can be achieved by either the intradermal or the subcutaneous route (Figs 3.4 and 3.5).

To establish a field block, cleanse the proposed

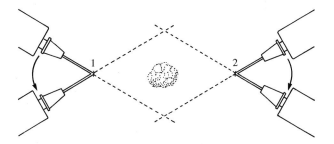

Fig. 3.6. Field block: rectilinear infiltration.

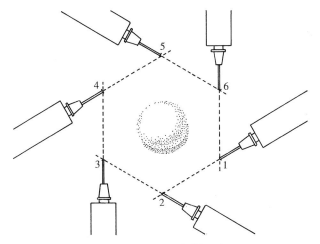

Fig. 3.7. Field block: polygonal infiltration.

Table 3.3. The advantages and disadvantages of intradermal and subcutaneous infiltration of local anaesthetic solutions

	Advantage	Disadvantage
Intradermal	Block achieved faster	Infiltration more painful
	Turgor of tissues facilitates incision, punch biopsy, etc.	Distortion of operation site
	Duration of block prolonged	
	Less risk of intravascular injection	
Subcutaneous	Infiltration less painful	Block slower to take effect
	Tissues less distorted	Effect wears off faster
		Greater risk of intravascular injection

operation site liberally with 70 per cent isopropyl alcohol. Plan the needle sites so that a minimum number of punctures are required for effective coverage of the area. For many procedures, a single entry at diagonal corners of a rectangle is sufficient (Fig. 3.6) but, for more extensive lesions, a polygonal approach may be required when all needle punctures after the first can be made through tissue which is already anaesthetized (Figure 3.7).

Nerve blocks

Nerve blocks enable anaesthetization of a whole area supplied by an accessible cutaneous nerve. They are particularly useful when local infiltration cannot be used, for example, on account of infection or where the operation site is particularly sensitive, for example, the tip of a finger. Blocks also enable smaller volumes of anaesthetic solution to be used although it is often necessary to use a stronger concentration of the agent to achieve satisfactory penetration of the nerve trunk.

Nerve blocks: 1. The hand

The median and the ulnar nerves are both readily accessible in the wrist for the induction of nerve block. The sensory fields involved are shown in Figs 3.8, 3.9 and the anatomical relations in Figure 3.10.

Median nerve

The median nerve enters the hand via the carpal tunnel (Fig. 3.10), a restricted space also containing the flexor tendons of the hand, bounded in front by the flexor retinaculum and behind by the small bones of the carpus. It lies almost centrally, below and slightly to the radial side of the palmaris longus tendon which, when present, is a useful landmark. To insert the block, identify the palmaris longus tendon by asking the patient to flex the fingers and wrist to the limit. Mark the injection site on the proximal transverse skin crease on the radial side of this tendon. Cleanse the skin with a spirit swab then, with the patient's wrist in the neutral position, insert the needle of a 2 ml syringe containing 2 per

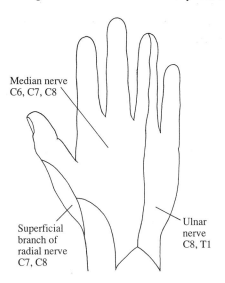

Fig. 3.8. Sensory innervation of hand: palmar surface.

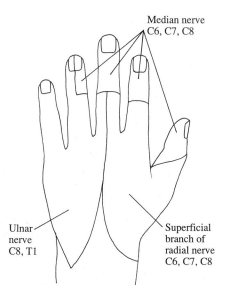

Fig. 3.9. Sensory innervation of hand: dorsal surface.

cent plain lignocaine at the marked point at an angle of approximately 30° to the forearm and for a distance of 10–15 mm. Pain in the median nerve distribution in the palm indicates that the needle has impinged on the nerve and it should be repositioned slightly. Remove the syringe from the needle and ask the patient to flex the fingers. The needle should not move, thus indicating that the flexor tendons are not involved. Replace the syringe and inject 1–2 ml lignocaine solution. There should be no resistance to the injection and the procedure should be painless. After 5–10 min paraesthesia and numbness of the blocked cutaneous area will develop.

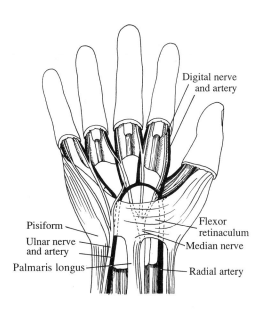

Fig. 3.10. Anatomy of median and ulnar nerves in the wrist (after Jamieson 1943).

Ulnar nerve

The ulnar nerve enters the hand (Fig. 3.10) superficial to the flexor retinaculum and lies just lateral (radial) to the pisiform bone. Mark this point on the distal transverse skin crease and, after cleansing the skin with a spirit swab, inject 1 ml 2 per cent plain lignocaine solution approximately 5 mm deep using a 25 guage (orange mount) needle. If the needle point causes paraesthesia in the ulnar sensory field, relocate it slightly before injecting. Again, anaesthesia should develop in 5–10 min.

Digital nerve

Appropriate for fingers, thumbs, and toes. Use 1 or 2 per cent plain lignocaine solution, **never** with added adrenalin. Proceed as follows.

Cleanse the whole digit with 0.5 per cent chlorhexidine in alcohol solution. Using an orange mount needle, inject 0.25 ml of 2 per cent *plain* lignocaine subcutaneously on either side of the dorsum of the digit opposite the mid-point of the proximal phalanx to anaesthetize the dorsal digital nerves (Fig. 3.11). Exchange the needle on the syringe for a blue mount needle and advance the point through the original injection sites on either side of the phalanx until the needle tip can be felt just distending the tissue on the volar surface of the digit (Fig. 3.12). Inject a further 0.75 ml of lignocaine on each side in the vicinity of the neurovascular bundle, withdrawing the syringe plunger slightly before injecting to ensure that a blood vessel has not been penetrated. The application of a tourniquet to the base of the digit will then expedite penetration of the nerve by the anaesthetic solution and also provide a blood-free field for the planned procedure. Snook (1971) has described an anterior approach to the palmar digital nerves which is appropriate when more proximal lesions on the fingers are to be approached.

Nerve blocks: 2. The foot

Similarly, nerve blocks can be performed on the foot, a useful technique where multiple lesions such as verrucae on the sole are to be treated and where, due to the thickness and fibrous nature of the dermis, local infiltration of anaesthetic solutions can often be very painful. The sensory fields of the posterior tibial and sural nerves are shown in Figs 3.13 and 3.14.

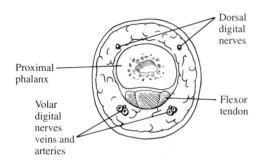

Fig. 3.11. Digital nerve block: transverse section of digit.

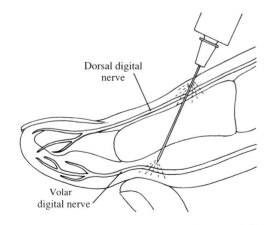

Fig. 3.12. Digital nerve block: lateral diagram of digital block.

Posterior tibial nerve

The posterior tibial nerve, on entering the foot, divides into the medial and lateral plantar nerves which supply the anterior two-thirds of the sole. It is accessible at the level of the ankle joint at a point midway between the posterior edge of the medial

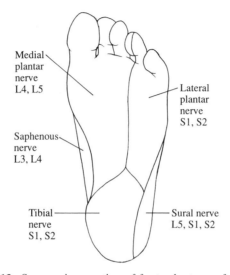

Fig. 3.13. Sensory innervation of foot: plantar surface.

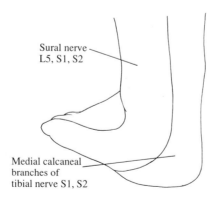

Fig. 3.14. Sensory innervation of foot: dorsal surface.

malleolus and the medial border of the tendo achillis (Fig. 3.15). The nerve lies immediately posterior to the posterior tibial artery and the pulsations provide a useful landmark. Palpate the artery and make a mark with a skin pencil approximately 5 mm posterior to it at the level of the medial malleolus. Cleanse the skin with an alcohol swab and, using a 25 gauge (orange mount) needle, inject 2–5 ml 2 per cent lignocaine at a depth of approximately 10 mm, aspirating first to ensure that the artery has not been entered.

Sural nerve

The sural nerve supplies the skin of the posterior third of the sole and the lateral border of the foot. It can be blocked at a point between the posterior edge of the lateral malleolus and the tendo achillis (Fig. 3.16) but it lies close to the short saphenous

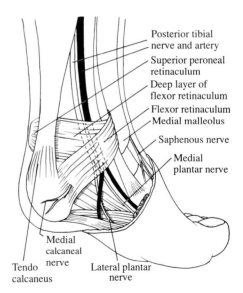

Fig. 3.15. Posterior tibial nerve: anatomy.

vein and its position is not entirely constant so the injection of lignocaine may need to be fanned antero-posteriorly, aspirating the while to ensure that the vein has not been entered. Three to six millilitres of 2 per cent lignocaine solution will usually be required.

Digital nerve block for toes
The principles outlined for the fingers should be employed.

A variety of additional nerve blocks are described by Auletta and Grekin (1991) relating in particular to the face and head but these are, perhaps, more applicable to formal plastic surgery than to the minor localized procedures encountered in general practice.

Regional nerve blocks
More extensive non-inhalational anaesthesia can be achieved by using relatively sophisticated techniques

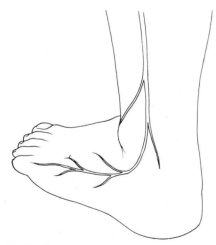

Fig. 3.16. Sural nerve: anatomy.

such as epidural block, brachial plexus block, and regional intravenous analgesia (Bier's block). These are the province of the specialist anaesthesiologist (Heath 1982) and are rarely, if ever, appropriate for the minor surgical procedures eligible for remuneration under the New Contract in general practice.

Amnalgesia
This technique, popular with some dental surgeons, may be useful for minor surgery for excessively apprehensive patients. It involves the cautious, continuous intravenous administration of a hypnotic, amnesia-inducing drug such as midazolam either alone or combined with an analgesic, for example, pethidine. The result is a relaxed, dozy, cooperative patient who has no subsequent recollection of the procedure. If this technique is used, it should **always** be supervised by a second practitioner and resuscitation equipment (see Chapter 1) should be to hand in case of need. The patient should starve for 4 h beforehand and should be accompanied home by a friend or relative. In the case of a female subject, a nurse should always be in attendance. On recovery, the patient should be instructed not to ride a bicycle or drive a car until the following day.

References
Auletta, M. J. and Grekin, R. C. (1991). *Local anaesthesia for dermatologic surgery*. Churchill Livingstone, New York.

Heath, M. L. (1982). Deaths after intravenous regional anaesthesia. *British Medical Journal*, **285**, 913–14.

Jamieson, E. B. (1977). *Illustrations of regional anatomy*. (9th edn). Churchill Livingstone, Edinburgh.

Kelly, D. A. and Henderson, A. M. (1983). Use of local anaesthetic drugs in hospital practice. *British Medical Journal*, **286**, 1783–4.

Snook, R. (1971). Minor surgery: local anaesthetics. *Update Plus*, **1**, 121–9.

Further reading
British National Formulary (1992). *15.2 Local anaesthesia*. British Medical Association and Royal Pharmaceutical Society of Great Britain, London.

Eriksson, E. (1980) *Illustrated handbook in local anaesthesia*, (2nd edn). Lloyd-Luke, London.

Robertson, J. F. R. and Muckart, D. J. J. (1985). Local anaesthesia of the great toe. *Journal of the Royal College of Surgeons of Edinburgh*, **30**, 237–8.

Scrimshire, J. A. (1989). Safe use of lignocaine. *British Medical Journal*, **298**, 1494.

Thomas, J. B. (1989). Anaesthesia In *Surgery for General Practitioners*, (ed. B. A. Maurice), pp. 76–80. Castle House Publications, Tunbridge Wells.

Wallace, W. A., Guardini, R., and Ellis, S. J. (1982). Standard intravenous regional analgesia. *British Medical Journal*, **285**, 554–6.

4 Medico-legal considerations

Introduction

The advantages for patients of minor surgical procedures being undertaken in the general practice setting are manifest; waiting times are usually short, the premises are often near their residence, the doctor is a familiar and trusted personality, and so on. In spite of the overt approval of authority by the introduction of specific remuneration for minor surgery, some practitioners remain hesitant about providing this service for fear of subsequent litigation, an anxiety sometimes reinforced by perusal of the annual reports of medical defence organizations. As in so many other fields of practice, success in this particular area depends not only on the skill of the doctor but also on good communication with the patient, so developing trust and confidence and, thus, minimizing the chance of medico-legal consequences. In this context, under common law, the patient has rights and the doctor has responsibilities which must both be acknowledged if, in the event of failure or complication of surgical procedures, such eventualities are to be avoided. These principles have been summarized in *A guide to consent for examination or treatment* which was published by the NHS Management Executive (1990) and some of the relevant points are detailed here.

The patient's rights

1. A patient has a right under common law to give or withhold consent to treatment. Thus, a doctor could face an action for assault if minor surgical procedures were undertaken without express consent, although this need not necessarily be in writing (see below).
2. Although there is no statutory legal requirement, patients are entitled to receive sufficient information regarding proposed treatment together with a résumé of the risks and the alternative options available so that they can make an informed decision before giving consent to proceed.
3. Care must always be taken to respect the patient's wishes. This is particularly important where the training of other health care professionals such as assistants and nurses is involved and specific consent in this respect should always be obtained as well.
4. As with any medical consultation and unless disclosure is deemed to be in the public interest, confidentiality is paramount and details of procedures must not be disclosed to third parties without the patient's knowledge and approval.

Advising the patient

Except in emergency situations, patients with conditions suitable for surgical treatment by general practitioners usually present themselves at routine consulting sessions when time is often limited and the actual treatment has to be deferred. However, the two immediate decisions that the doctor should make at this point are:

(1) what is the probable diagnosis?;
(2) am I competent to deal with this condition or would the patient be better served by referral to a colleague with more experience either within the practice or to a hospital specialist?

Having decided that referral is not necessary, the remainder of the consultation should be utilized for informing the patient about the condition and its management. The following points should be addressed:

(1) the diagnosis, aetiology, and prognosis of the condition;
(2) the nature of the surgical procedure proposed;
(3) when and where it will be performed;
(4) how long it will take;
(5) the intended method of analgesia;
(6) arrangements for aftercare;
(7) whether absence from work or school will be necessary;
(8) possible complications, for example, pain, bruising, scarring;
(9) has the patient further questions?

When these details have been explained to the patient's satisfaction, verbal consent should be obtained (see below) and an appointment made for the procedure to be undertaken. The availability of a minor surgery information leaflet (for example, Appendix A) for the patient will provide confirmation of the arrangements made.

Obtaining consent

Valid consent for treatment in medical practice takes two main forms: it may be either implied or express, the latter obtained orally or in writing. Implied consent may be dictated by circumstance, for example, when a patient keeps an appointment for a specific procedure to be undertaken or undresses to expose a lesion for removal. Express consent, on the other hand, is given when the patient confirms acceptance of treatment in clear and explicit terms, either orally (preferably, but not necessarily, in front of a witness) or in writing. In general, consent for minor surgical procedures should be express rather than implied. Oral consent is adequate for the great majority of procedures undertaken in general practice but written consent should be obtained in cases where there is substantial risk of complication or where there is a communication difficulty with the patient. In the case of treatment of young persons under the age of 16 years consent should ideally be obtained from a parent or other responsible adult although a minor can in fact give informed consent to a simple procedure (for example, suture of a superficial wound) provided the doctor is satisfied that the patient understands the true nature, purpose, and potential hazards of the procedure. On the other hand, under the terms of the Children Act 1989, parents can give valid consent, where a procedure is clearly in the child's best interests, to treatment of a minor who actively dissents. In instances where a patient is over the age of 16 years but not competent to give consent (by virtue, for example, of mental impairment), then consent of a parent or guardian should be sought but again this is not mandatory in law provided the surgeon is satisfied that the treatment is in the best interests of the patient. If general anaesthesia is to be used, written consent should always be obtained from the patient (or in the case of a minor, the parent or person acting *in loco parentis*). When written consent is obtained, the document should always be retained in the patient's medical records. Specimen consent forms are shown in Appendix B. The whole question of consent to treatment is concisely dealt with in a small monograph published by the Medical Defence Union (Anon. 1992) and available to non-members at a nominal charge.

The doctor's responsibilities
Training
In law, doctors are required to demonstrate that they have provided patients with a standard of care not inferior to that generally provided by colleagues in similar circumstances. However, it has been stated that if a doctor fails to exercise the skill which he has or claims to have (for example, in minor surgery), he is in breach of his duty of care and is, therefore, negligent (Donaldson 1980). Thus, whilst this handbook aims to give guidance on the basic principles of minor surgery and on some specific procedures in more detail, doctors without previous experience in the discipline should initially perform minor operations under the supervision of an experienced colleague until competence is assured and confidence has developed. Indeed, a case can be made for subspecialization in minor surgery by one or more interested partners in a practice, at least with regard to the more complicated or extensive procedures illustrated and this is not at variance with the regulations concerning remuneration (see Chapter 6).

Accreditation
The criteria for accreditation for minor surgery in the National Health Service are summarized in Chapter 6. Doctors need to show that they have undertaken specific training for or have regularly practised the required skills during the five years before application. Doctors who do not fulfil the required criteria *ab initio* may achieve accreditation by attendance at a recognized theoretical course on minor surgery lasting at least 1 day (6 h) and by showing evidence of practical experience as recommended by their Regional General Practice Education Committee. Guidelines on training and required facilities for minor surgery have been issued to Local Medical Committees, RCGP faculties, and Regional Advisors in General Practice (DHSS 1991) whence further advice may be obtained. According to the regulations at the time of writing, doctors providing minor surgery services were expected to be competent in performing all the procedures listed in the schedule although, in some circumstances, injection of varicose veins and haemorrhoids might be excluded.

Surgical procedure
The avowed purpose of this volume is to emphasize good practice and to highlight approved surgical techniques. However, to avoid medico-legal consequences, the following points should be always borne in mind.

1. Doctors should always be aware of their personal limitations in the field and respect the vernacular aphorism: 'If in doubt, don't!'. In particular, whenever possible, avoid operating in 'high risk' areas of the body (see Chapter 5).
2. Bearing in mind the duty of care to the patient, do not, on the grounds of time or expedience, deviate from established routines by taking short cuts. In particular, risk most often relates to inadequate sterilization of equipment or failure to employ approved aseptic techniques.
3. Always send excised tissue for histological examination, properly labelled, and with full clinical details. Ensure, too, that the reports are reviewed and that appropriate action is taken; this is the basis of efficient clinical audit. Whimster and Leonard (1991) have drawn attention to a number of studies identifying substandard performance in

general practice due to inaccurate clinical diagnosis, failure to refer specimens, inadequate excision, poor fixation, and so on.

4. Unless the technique dictates otherwise, it is best to operate with the patient recumbent, thus avoiding actual or potential injury from vasovagal attacks or fainting.

5. Except for the simplest consulting room procedures, such as uncomplicated steroid injections, always endeavour to have a nursing assistant in attendance. Not only can they give psychologial support to the patient and practical assistance to the surgeon but can also serve as an unofficial witness to the procedures undertaken. For this reason, it may also be a sensible precaution to enter their name in the Minor Operations Register (see below).

Records
Clinical notes
As with any other doctor–patient contact, concise and accurate records are of the essence. A note should be made in the patient's NHS records at the time of the procedure regarding both consent and details of the operation performed. Histology reports, in particular, should also be included. Any subsequent complication should be recorded together with details of its management and relevant information given to the patient. These notes will, of course, follow the patient to subsequent medical attendants and provide the definitive record of treatment should legal proceedings ensue.

The minor operations register
It is also advisable to maintain a lasting record of all minor operations undertaken and these registers

should be retained within the practice for as long as possible. Minimum data should be recorded in a hardback notebook kept in the treatment area and should include:

(1) date and time of operation;
(2) patient identification, that is, name, sex, and date of birth;
(3) surgeon's name;
(4) name of assistant or nurse in attendance;
(5) nature of the procedure completed;
(6) type of anaesthesia/analgesia used;
(7) tissue sent for histology (if any);
(8) notes, for example, complications, variation from routine methods, etc.

A specimen page is shown in Appendix D of Chapter 6 and it should be the responsibility of the treatment room nurse to ensure that all procedures are recorded therein, whether or not these are included in the schedule of items approved for remuneration.

Miscellaneous considerations
General health and safety
It is important that practices, whether undertaking minor surgery or not, have a documented policy for the care and protection of staff (Ellis 1987). The law also demands that written records are kept of any accidental injury befalling staff and that serious accidents are reported to the Health and Safety Executive. As far as treatment room procedures are concerned, these requirements are concisely summarized in Appendix 7 of the BMA handbook *Sterilisation of instruments and control of cross infection* (Morgan 1989).

Disposal of clinical waste
Doctors, as generators of potentially hazardous clinical waste, have a duty under the Health and Safety at Work Act 1974, to ensure that such waste is collected, stored and disposed of safely and in accordance with regulations (DoE 1992). Equipment appropriate to this purpose has been described in Chapter 1 and, again, the whole matter is concisely dealt with in Section 6 of the BMA handbook referred to above (Morgan 1989).

Product liability
Consumer protection law (Consumer Protection Act 1987, Part 1) requires a manufacturer to ensure that his product is up to standard and fit for its intended purpose. The supplier (user) of that product then has a responsibility to identify the manufacturer if damage is caused by a defect in the product. If this cannot be done, then liability may rest with the supplier (user). Doctors become suppliers when they dispense any product to a patient or use a product in the course of treatment (Dando 1991). To avoid liability it is thus essential for the doctor to know the name of the manufacturer of that product. As far as minor surgical procedures are concerned, it is therefore necessary to record manufacturers' names, the source of supplies, batch numbers, dates of purchase, etc. and to check expiry dates of degradable products before use. Furthermore, as far as equipment is concerned, product liability may shift from the manufacturer to the user if the former can show that the equipment has not been used or maintained in accordance with the instructions. Doctors should therefore ensure that a responsible member of their staff, perhaps the nursing sister in charge of the treatment room, ensures that these requirements are fulfilled and that appropriate records are kept. Finally, doctors and treatment

room nurses should be aware that the inappropriate recycling of single-use products could render them liable in the event of consequent damage or injury to a patient.

Quality control and audit

In practices where minor surgery makes a significant contribution to patient care, results should be monitored by regular audit. In addition to the analysis, for fiscal reasons, of the procedures undertaken (see Chapter 6), a number of relevant indicators such as histology reports, concordance of pathological with clinical diagnoses, and complication rates (for example, the incidence of wound dehiscence or secondary infection) could be assessed. Production of the results of regular reviews of this type and their inclusion in the practice annual report would, in the event of litigation, provide evidence of a professional approach to the services offered to patient.

Conclusion

Recognition of personal limitations, attention to detail, and good communication with patients will greatly reduce the chance of subsequent litigation. The medico-legal aspects of minor surgery are succinctly covered in another Medical Defence Union monograph (Dando 1991).

References

Anon (1992). *Consent to treatment*. The Medical Defence Union Ltd, London.

Dando, P. (1991). *Medico-legal aspects of minor surgery*. The Medical Defence Union Ltd, London.

Department of the Environment (1992). *Waste management—the duty of care. A Code of Practice*. HMSO, London.

Department of Health and Social Security (1991). *Minor surgery in general practice*. Guidelines by the General Medical Services Committee and the Royal College of General Practitioners in collaboration with the Royal College of Surgeons of England and the Royal College of Surgeons of Edinburgh and the Joint Committee on Postgraduate Training for General Practice, DHSS, London.

Donaldson, L. J. (1980). *Whitehouse -v- Jordan [1980].* 1 All ER 650–8, 662.

Ellis, N. (1987). *Employing staff*, (2nd edn). British Medical Journal Books, British Medical Association, London.

Morgan, D. (ed.) (1989). *A code of practice for sterilisation of instruments and control of cross infection*. British Medical Association, London.

National Health Service Management Executive (1990). *A guide to consent for examination or treatment*. DHSS, London.

Whimster, W. F. and Leonard, R. A. (1991). Surgical pathology and general practice. *British Medical Journal*, **303**, 1149–50.

Appendix A: consent form

CONSENT FORM

For medical or dental investigation, treatment or operation

Health Authority ....

Hospital ....

Unit Number ....

Patient's Surname ....

Other Names ....

Date of Birth ....

Sex: *(please tick)*   Male ____   Female ____

DOCTORS OR DENTISTS   *(This part to be completed by doctor or dentist. See notes on the reverse)*

Type of operation, investigation or treatment for which written evidence of consent is considered appropriate

I confirm that I have explained the operation, investigation or treatment, and such appropriate options as are available and the type of anaesthetic, if any (general/local/sedation) proposed, to the patient in terms which in my judgement are suited to the understanding of the patient and/or to one of the parents or guardians of the patient.

Signature ....   Date ..... / ..... / .....

Name of doctor or dentist ....

PATIENT/PARENT/GUARDIAN

1. Please read this form and the notes overleaf very carefully.

2. If there is anything that you don't understand about the explanation, or if you want more information, you should ask the doctor or dentist.

3. Please check that all the information on the form is correct. If it is, and you understand the explanation, then sign the form.

I am the patient/parent/guardian *(delete as necessary)*

I agree ▪ to what is proposed which has been explained to me by the doctor/dentist named on this form.

▪ to the use of the type of anaesthetic that I have been told about.

I understand ▪ that the procedure may not be done by the doctor/dentist who has been treating me so far.

▪ that any procedure in addition to the investigation or treatment described on this form will only be carried out if it is necessary and in my best interests and can be justified for medical reasons.

I have told ▪ the doctor or dentist about the procedures listed below I would **not** wish to be carried out without my having the opportunity to consider them first.

....
....

Signature ....

Name ....

Address ....

(if not the patient)

NOTES TO:

Doctors, Dentists

A patient has a legal right to grant or withhold consent prior to examination or treatment. Patients should be given sufficient information, in a way they can understand, about the proposed treatment and the possible alternatives. Patients must be allowed to decide whether they will agree to the treatment and they may refuse or withdraw consent to treatment at any time. The patient's consent to treatment should be recorded on this form (further guidance is given in HC(90)22: A Guide to Consent for Examination or Treatment).

Patients

■ The doctor or dentist is here to help you. He or she will explain the proposed treatment and what the alternatives are. You can ask any questions and seek further information. You can refuse the treatment.

■ You may ask for a relative, or friend, or a nurse to be present.

■ Training doctors and dentists and other health professionals is essential to the continuation of the health service and improving the quality of care. Your treatment may provide an important opportunity for such training, where necessary under the careful supervision of a senior doctor or dentist.

▨ You may, however, decline to be involved in the formal training of medical, dental and other students without this adversely affecting your care and treatment.

Appendix B: form to be used for patients unable to consent because of mental disorder

Medical or dental treatment of a patient who is unable to consent because of mental disorder

Health Authority ....

Hospital ....

Unit Number ....

Patient's Surname ....

Other Names ....

Date of Birth ....

Sex: *(please tick)*   Male ____   Female ____

NOTE:

It is the personal responsibility of any doctor or dentist proposing to treat a patient to determine whether the patient has capacity to give a valid consent.

It is good practice to consult relatives and others who are concerned with the care of the patient. Sometimes consultation with a specialist or specialists will be required.

The form should be signed by the doctor or dentist who carries out the treatment.

DOCTORS/DENTISTS

Describe investigation, operation or treatment proposed.

(Complete this part of the form)

In my opinion .... is not capable of giving consent to treatment. In my opinion the treatment proposed is in his/her best interests and should be given.

The patient's next of kin have/have not been so informed.   *(delete as necessary)*

Date: ....

Signature: ....

Name of doctor or dentist who is providing treatment:

....

Appendix C: minor operations—information for patients

MINOR OPERATIONS - INFORMATION FOR PATIENTS

INTRODUCTION

Our Minor Operating Clinics are held in the Outpatient Department of the Chiltern Hospital on Monday afternoon and Tuesday mornings. Minor operations are normally performed either by Dr. John Wilkinson or Dr. Carole Floyer, who specialises in dermatological surgery. You may eat and drink normally prior to your visit.

Your minor operation will take between ten to thirty minutes and you will be able to go home directly the procedure has been completed. If you feel at all nervous, it is a good idea to bring a friend or relative for moral support. All young people under the age of 16 must be accompanied.

Types of Procedures carried out at the Minor Operations Clinic

1. **Excisions:** This means the complete removal of a lump, mole or blemish. The skin will be repaired with stitches to leave as neat a scar as possible. The piece of skin removed will normally be sent to a laboratory for confirmation of the diagnosis.

2. **Biopsies:** This means taking a small sample of skin to send to the laboratory for testing. This test will help to make an accurate diagnosis of your problem. We frequently perform a biopsy on rashes or on large lesions that are too big to remove completely. The skin wound will be very small, usually about one centimetre long, but will need closing with sutures.

3. **Minor procedures:** These include simple techniques such as curettage (scraping off), cautery (burning), cryotherapy (freezing) or electrodiathermy (coagulation). These procedures usually result in small superficial wounds similar to grazes or light burns. They do not require stitches, but may need (daily) cleaning with dilute antiseptic and covering with a non-occlusive plaster for a few days until they dry up and heal. This can be done by yourself at home.

CLINIC ROUTINES

Consent Form

You will be asked to sign a consent form (unless you are under 16 when a parent or guardian must sign). This form indicates to us that you are aware of the procedure that we are going to carry out. Most minor operations need local anaesthetic (pain killer) to numb the area. This will be injected just under the area to be treated. General anaesthetic, the type that puts you to sleep, is never used in Out-patients.

When you are asked to sign this form, please tell us about any/all pills, tablets, medicines or sprays that you are taking. Also tell us if you have any allergies.

Undressing

You will be asked to remove enough clothing so that we can clearly see the part of your body involved.

Marking

The area of skin to be removed will often be marked with ink.

Operating Couch

Apart from exceptional circumstances such as immobility or breathlessness, all patients will be treated lying down on an operating couch. This makes the operation easier and allows us to use a good overhead light to see clearly.

Local Anaesthetic

The anaesthetic is injected just under the skin around the area to be removed. It causes a sharp sting which lasts 5 - 10 seconds. The operation will then be pain free. Please let us know if you feel any discomfort or have previously experienced any difficulty with local anaesthetic.

The follwing information is for those interested in the type of anaesthetic used. 1% or 2% Lignocaine combined with 1 in 80,000 Adrenaline is usually used. This combination provides very rapid numbness and also some vasoconstriction (closing off of small blood vessels) which helps to reduce bleeding. In some areas such as fingers and toes the adrenaline is omitted from the anaesthetic. This is done to prevent any circulation problems.

Surgery

Will be performed by doctors will particular experience in Dermatological Surgery.

A nurse will be in attendance.

Stitches

Most minor operations will be very small and the skin will be repaired using a few skin stitches. The stitches will not be dissolvable and will need removing.

In a few cases where the wound is larger, we may need to use some deep dissolvable stitches in addition to the skin stitches. This is done to give strength to the repair and also to help draw the skin edges nearer together.

Stitches will be left in place for between 1 and 2 weeks. As a rough guide, in quick healing areas, e.g. the face, they will be removed after one week. Stitches in areas overlying large muscles, e.g. back, thighs, will be removed after 2 weeks.

Strapping

All stitched wounds will be well strapped up with special dressings. We advise you to leave our dressings in place if possible until the stitches have been removed. After the stitches have been removed, we will re-apply strapping which should be left in place for a similar length of time.

The newly healed wound takes several weeks to gain strength and care during this time will improve the final appearance of the scar.

Sports and strenuous activities may stretch the scar and should be avoided for a few weeks.

Stitch Removal

You will be asked to make an appointment for your stitches to be removed at the hospital. You and your G.P. will both be notified of the results of the laboratory test (histology). This normally takes ten to fourteen days. For many small lesions no follow-up appointment will be necessary so long as histology confirms the expected diagnosis and so long as everything heals satisfactorily. Following diagnostic biopsy or when further treatment is required you will have been asked to make a follow-up appointment with the doctor who referred you for surgery.

When no follow-up is needed, it is often worth revisiting your own General Practioner after three months so that he can check that everything has healed satisfactorily.

PROBLEMS THAT CAN OCCUR

Between us we perform several thousand operations a year and in the vast majority of these there are no complications or side effects. There are, however, a few problems which very occasionally occur and we feel you should be fully informed of the minor difficulties that can sometimes happen.

Inflammation

Normally a slight redness around the stitches. This usually settles down on its own when the stitches have been removed.

Infection

Sometimes the treated area can become infected. This gives rise to pain, swelling and redness or there may be some pus present. If this happens, you should contact our nurses so that they can check the wound and arrange for our resident Medical Officer to provide antibiotics (if necessary) or you should visit your own G.P. and he will decide whether a course of antibiotics is necessary.

Bleeding

Even a small operation around the eyes is likely to cause some bruising and may give rise to a "black eye" In other areas bleeding is less likely but can occur, especially following larger operations. This may give rise to bruising.

Very occasionally a wound may bleed sufficiently to need re-stitching or a small blood vessel may need recoagulating. Again, we, or our resident Medical Officer, can be contacted through the nurses in Out-patients. Alternatively, seek advice from your G.P. or an Accident and Emergency Department if you are away from home. Five or ten minutes of simple pressure is usually enough to stop most bleeding. If the affected area is a limb, elevation will also help.

Fainting

A few people feel faint or sick during or after an operation. If you let us know how you are feeling we will raise your feet and give you some oxygen. This will make you feel a lot better. Patients who have fainted will be kept in the department until they feel better and be checked before going home.

Anaesthetic Problems

1. Palpitations can occur in a few people. The local anaesthetic and adrenaline can give rise to a feeling of rapid heart beat. If this happens, a few minutes' rest before returning home is advised. The feeling of palpitation is caused by the adrenaline in the local anaesthetic and can be avoided if you are aware of the problem. If this has ever happened, please let us know.

2. Allergy to the local anaesthetic is extremely rare indeed. We have only had one case in the last 10 years. If you have had problems with local anaesthetic, please let us know.

Scarring

It is impossile to remove anything without leaving a scar. As a general rule, the length of the scar is three times the width of the lump to be removed.

1. Stretching of scar: A wide stretched scar can occur especially if strapping has been removed too soon or activities that stretch the scar resumed too early. Excisions overlying large muscle groups and near joints are more likely to stretch.

2. Hypertrophic or Keloid scars: This is an over-reaction to the fibrous tissue/scar tissue in your skin. It does not happen immediately but develops a few weeks after surgery. It is more common in scars which have not been sufficiently immobilised. Keloid scars are due to an individual/inherent tendency to form scar tissue and are more common on the front of the chest, upper arms and upper back. They can occur in anyone but the problem is more common amongst Afro-Caribbean skin types. If you have had any previous problem with thickened scars, please let us know.

3. Bursting of the wound: This is extremely rare. The most likely time for this to occur is just after the stitches have been removed or if the wound becomes infected. The wound may then require re-suturing. Special care and good strapping for the days just after the sutures have been removed will reduce the risk of this happening.

Nerve Damage

1. Sensation: When the area of skin to be removed is quite large, it may be necessary to cut some small nerves in the skin. This type of nerve deals with the feeling of touch. This means you may have a small area of numbness around or just beyond the wound. Although substantial recovery may occur in time, you can be left with a small permanent area of numbness.

2. Movement: At our Minor Operations Clinics we have never caused any damage to nerves that deal with movement. There are, however, certain areas, especially on the face, where deep surgery could cause damage to nerves responsible for movement. We restrict surgery in these areas but there is always a small risk that nerves may be abnormally placed or hidden in among a tumour and could therefore be damaged by surgery.

Any surgery will involve some small risk. When there is a malignancy the benefits will obviously always outweigh the risks. Where a biopsy will help to make a diagnosis, this is also true. For cosmetic operations it is however sensible to be sure that the scar is going to be more acceptable than the lesion to be removed and other inherent risks of surgery will also have to be taken into account.

5 Basic principles of minor surgery

Although the procedures detailed in Chapter 7 are illustrated as comprehensively as space allows, many assume a basic knowledge of simple surgical techniques. Experience as a house officer in a surgical firm is a mandatory requirement for medical registration in the United Kingdom but two recent studies (Chew 1991; Pringle *et al.* 1991) reveal a singular lack of confidence in the performance of simple procedures by GP trainees and question the adequacy of postgraduate instruction in the hospital setting. Cox *et al.* (1992) suggest an audit process to redress the prevailing situation and this chapter summarizes the simple skills appropriate to the procedures listed later.

Incision technique

As an example of a basic incision technique, the removal of a superficial lesion such as a pigmented naevus or dermatofibroma can be used (Fig. 5.1). The principles to be adopted are as follows.

1. Plan the operation. In most cases a fusiform (spindle-shaped) incision circumscribing the lesion is appropriate. The long axis should be aligned with existing skin creases and wrinkle lines or, in the absence of the these, be guided by Langer's hypothetical lines (Gibson 1978) (Appendix A). Bear in mind that the lines of maximum tension will vary in the vicinity of joints and plan the incision so that tension is not further increased when the free edges of the resulting wound are approximated.

2. Mark the proposed incisions using a skin pencil. A fibre-tip pen may be used although the mark tends to be removed by alcohol-based skin cleansers. Gentian violet solution, once popular, should not be used; it is now thought that it may be carcinogenic. To ensure neat closure, the long axis of the incision should measure not less than three times that of the transverse diameter.

3. Infiltrate the local anaesthetic solution (see Chapter 3) and test that it has taken effect, then make the required incisions as follows.
   (a) Tension the skin at right angles to the line of incision using the thumb and forefinger of the free hand.
   (b) Make the incision holding the knife at right angles to the skin surface. To facilitate accurate closure in hairy areas, however, the incision plane should be parallel to the emergent angle of the hair follicles (Figs 5.2 and 5.3).
   (c) Try to incise the corium completely with a single confident stroke so that the tip of the blade penetrates to the fatty subcutaneous layer but not so far as the deep fascia; bear in mind that the thickness and density of the skin varies considerably in different parts of the body.
   (d) Avoid 'fish-tailing' at the apices of the wound which will complicate accurate closure (Fig. 5.4).

NB. There are certain areas of the body where major vital structures (nerves, arteries, veins,

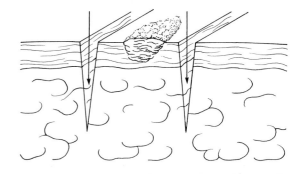

Fig. 5.2. The cutaneous incision (cross-section).

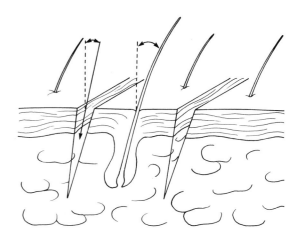

Fig. 5.3. The cutaneous incision (hairy area) (cross-section).

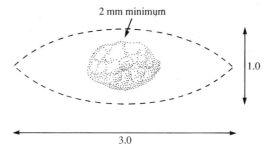

2 mm minimum

1.0

3.0

Fig. 5.1. The fusiform excision plan.

tendons, etc.) lie relatively close to the surface and excisions in these localities should be approached with considerable caution. Danger areas are, in particular, the pre-auricular area of the face, the front and side of the neck, the axilla, the wrist, the inguinal and femoral triangles, the popliteal fossa, the palmar surface of the fingers, and the anterior aspect of the ankle.

Excision for histological examination

Excision biopsy is a common indication for the removal of superficial lesions; the following points of technique should be adopted.

1. A narrow strip of normal skin (2 mm) should be included on either side of the lesion. To ensure complete excision, be certain that the incisions are made outside the lines marked.
2. Tissue should be removed with minimum traumatization to facilitate microscopic examination; handling can be reduced by lifting it out of the wound with a fine skin hook or silk suture through the apex of the specimen rather than by gripping it with toothed forceps (Fig. 5.5a and b).
3. Separate intradermal lesions by blunt-tipped scissor dissection through the adipose layer (separate and snip) (Fig. 5.6).
4. Immediately on removal, place the specimen in a vessel containing 10 per cent formalin in normal saline solution for transfer to the laboratory.

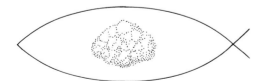

Fig. 5.4. The 'fish-tail' fault.

5. Ensure that the card accompanying the specimen includes the following information:
   (a) patient identification, including sex and date of birth;
   (b) data and time of operation;
   (c) original site of lesion;
   (d) provisional diagnosis;
   (e) examination required.

Haemostasis

Bleeding is rarely a problem with the superficial procedures usually carried out in general practice. However, if it seems to be excessive, one or more of the following measures can be employed.

1. Firm pressure with a gauze swab for 2 min by the clock.
2. Reposture the patient, for example, if

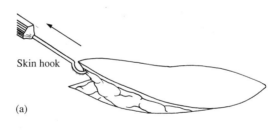

Skin hook

(a)

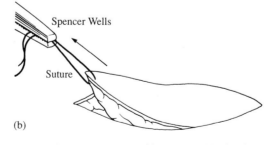

Spencer Wells

Suture

(b)

Fig. 5.5. Specimen elevation (a) using a skin hook, (b) using a suture.

bleeding is on the face, sit the patient up, if on the leg, elevate the limb.
3. Irrigate the wound with a few drops of lignocaine solution containing adrenaline which is often to hand after initiating local analgesia.
4. Use a haemostatic solution such as aluminium chloride 20 per cent in 70 per cent isopropyl alcohol applied with a sterile throat swab. Monsel's solution (basic ferric sulphate) is also effective but may stain the skin. Silver nitrate or trichloroacetic acid should not be used on account of their corrosive properties.

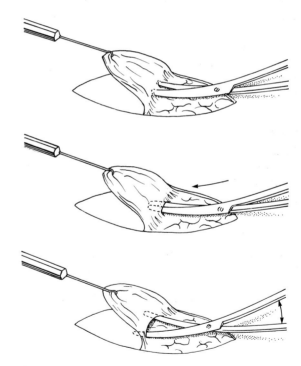

Fig. 5.6. Blunt dissection: scissor technique (separate and snip)

5. Small bleeding points may be crushed for a few seconds with fine mosquito forceps.
6. If bleeding still persists, tie off the arteriole with fine (4/0) chromic catgut.
7. If diathermy apparatus (for example, Hyfrecator) is available, touch bleeding points with the monopolar tip or bipolar coagulation forceps.

Wound Closure

The primary objective is that the wound should heal by first intention and leave a fine linear scar that, in older subjects at least, may be mistaken for a wrinkle or skin crease. This aim is especially important for female patients and where procedures are undertaken on visible areas of the body, the face in particular.

Suture Materials
Absorbable
Used for the approximation of deep tissues, the suturing of wounds on mucous membranes (for example, mouth or vagina) and for haemostasis; although synthetic absorbable sutures are now available, only those made from chromic catgut are listed in the Drug Tariff (2.0 and 3.5 metric gauge, see Appendix B).

Non-absorbable
Used for skin closure; made of monofilament nylon (Ethilon) or polypropylene (Prolene); available on the Drug Tariff in a variety of weights (0.7, 1.5, 2.0, and 3.5 metric gauge, see Appendix B). Braided silk (Mersilk) sutures (1.5, 2.0, and 3.0 metric gauge) are also available. Since they cause a greater tissue reaction than monofilament synthetics and leave

more obvious suture marks, their use should be limited to areas such as flexures and the perineum where pricking from the suture ends has to be avoided.

Needles
Needles bonded to the suture filaments come in various styles and sizes. Atraumatic (round-bodied) needles are used for subcutaneous repair and mucous membranes. Cutting (triangular in cross-section) needles are used for tougher tissues, in particular, the skin. Reverse cutting needles should be used for suturing close to tissue margins or where sutures are unavoidably under tension; the filament is then less likely to cut out. Again, a variety of needle sizes and forms (curved and half-circle) are available. Straight cutting needles, which are useful for continuous subcuticular sutures (Fig. 5.9) are not available in the Drug Tariff.

Suturing technique
Simple skin closure
This method, which is appropriate for superficial lacerations and incisions, is illustrated in Fig. 5.7. Monofilament synthetic sutures should be used of the finest possible gauge, especially for the face. Needle entry and exit points should be equidistant from skin edges and evenly spaced along the length of the wound. Leave tails approximately 5 mm long and lay the knots all to the same side of the incision for a neat final result.

For longer incisions, the 'halving' technique (Fig. 5.8) will ensure a symmetrical result.

Where the wound does not gape unduly, neat closure can be achieved by the use of a single monofilament subcuticular 'zigzag' suture (Fig. 5.9) from end to end.

Finally, where there is neither gaping of nor undue tension on the wound edges, sterile adhesive skin closure strips (Steri-strips) or enbucrilate tissue adhesive (Histoacryl Blue, now also avaialble on FP10) may suffice, thus obviating the need for painful infiltration of local anaesthetic solution. Ensure, however, that the skin surfaces are

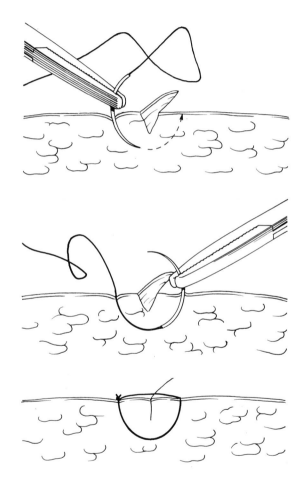

Fig. 5.7. Simple suturing technique.

completely free from moisture and grease or they may not adhere effectively.

Deeper wounds

Unless subcutaneous tissues (particularly fat) are properly secured and dead spaces obliterated, haematomata may form or infection occur and cause

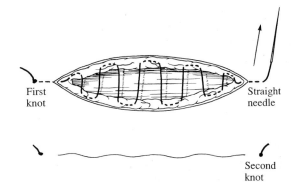

Fig. 5.9. Subcuticular closure technique.

consequent wound dehiscence when the sutures are removed. There are a number of ways in which this can be prevented.

1. Use interrupted deep sutures (absorbable) with inverted knots, then close the skin by one of the methods described above (Fig. 5.10).
2. Use vertical mattress sutures (Fig. 5.11) of monofilament material. The superficial bites should be within 1–2 mm of the skin edges, the deep bites approximately 7.5 mm. To ensure that the cavity of the wound is property opposed, it is best to insert the deep bite first. The disadvantage of mattress sutures is that they result in a double row of needle-puncture marks after removal.
3. Use interrupted 'figure of eight' monofilament sutures (Fig. 5.12). The

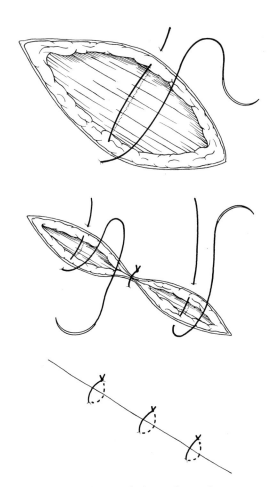

Fig. 5.8. The 'halving' technique of suturing.

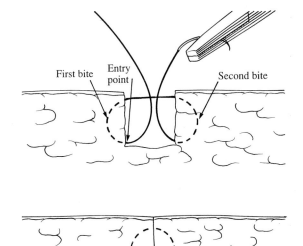

Fig. 5.10. Deep suture with inverted knot.

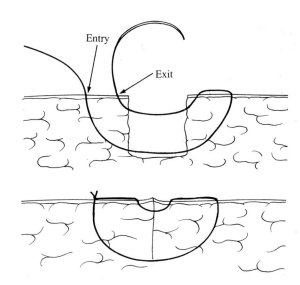

Fig. 5.11. The vertical mattress suture.

principle of closure is similar to that of mattress sutures but only single needle-puncture marks result so they may be cosmetically more acceptable although suture removal is sometimes more difficult.

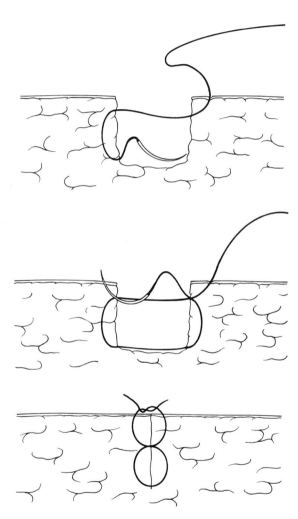

Fig. 5.12. The 'figure of eight' suture.

Knots

All knots, whether deep or superficial, should be of the flat (square) variety, that is, 'reefs' not 'grannies'. The latter slip, the former will not, as boy scouts and girl guides will remember! Always add a third throw for extra security. When synthetic materials (Ethilon, Prolene) are being used and the wound edges are approximated under tension, a

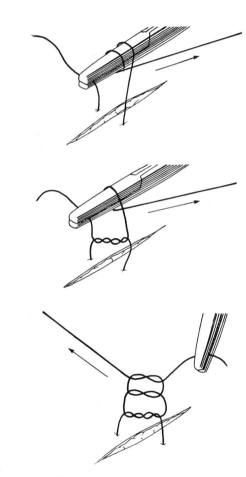

Fig. 5.13. Tying and laying knots.

double hitch for the first throw (Fig. 5.13) will prevent slippage before the second throw is taken.

Deep sutures should be cut close to the knot and non-absorbable sutures (Ethilon, Prolene, silk) should have 5–10 mm tails to facilitate identification and removal. The uninitiated should practice suturing and knot-tying one-handed or with instruments, on old leather gloves or pieces of discarded neoprene wet suits before embarking on real life practice! For the more affluent, simulator kits are now commercially available (Chapter 1, Appendix A).

Emergency technique

Doctors do not always carry sterile packs of instruments in their medical bags so some means of improvised suturing may occasionally be necessary. Scalp wounds, for example, may, after cleansing with soap and water and achieving haemostasis by gentle pressure, be closed by twisting a few hairs together on either side of the laceration, then tying them across the wound (Fig. 5.14). On non-hairy areas, opposition of wound edges can be achieved by the use of a sterile hypodermic needle through which a filament can be threaded, then tied after withdrawal of the needle (Fig. 5.15).

Dressings

'An ideal dressing protects the wound physically, keeps it warm and moist, assists the removal of exudate, encourages healing and reduces the likelihood of infection' (Anon 1991). In fact, in the case of clean surgical wounds, which heal by first intention, a minimalist approach with regard to dressings can be observed.

1. In hairy situations like the scalp or where bandaging is difficult or where cosmetic

considerations apply (for example, on the face) hydron copolymer 3 per cent in acetone/ethyl acetate 20 per cent aerosol (Opsite spray) is useful and permits the patient to wash the area prior to suture removal. Ensure that the surrounding skin is dry and mask off sensitive areas, such as the eye, before application.

2. Small wounds up to 2 cm long may be protected by semi-permeable plastic waterproof sterile wound dressings (Airstrip) which are available in a variety of sizes.

3. Larger areas may be covered by perforated film absorbent dressing (Melolin, 5 cm × 5 cm) held in position with permeable synthetic adhesive tape (Micropore) or, in situations where a water-resistant dressing is required, by impermeable tape (Blenderm) or a semi-permeable film dressing (Bioclusive, Opsite Flexigrid, Tegaderm) which are available in packs containing ten 10 cm × 12 cm pieces that can be cut to required sizes.

4. In some situations (for example, in the vicinity of joints) a non-adhesive dressing may best be held in place by cotton conforming bandages (Crinx, Kling, Slinky) or elastic net surgical tubular stockingette (Netelast, Texagrip, Tubigrip).

5. Dressings for wounds on fingers and toes are most conveniently secured by cotton yarn tubular bandage (Tubegauz) which is available in a number of sizes with matched applicator frames. Since a twisting action is required for the application of tubular bandages, it is important to avoid a tourniquet effect at the base of the digit.

6. When raw areas (for example, a toenail bed) are being dressed, a sterile gauze dressing impregnated with soft paraffin (Jelonet) is appropriate.

7. If the dressing is required incorporating an antiseptic agent, povidine-iodine (Inadine) or chlorhexidine (Bactigras) impregnated gauzes are available.

A selection of wound dressings prescribable on FP10 is shown in Appendix C.

Redressing of wounds after minor surgical procedures should be at the doctor's or nurse's discretion. Suffice it to say that dressings should not be changed routinely prior to suture removal but, if there is any evidence of complications (*quod vide*), it is prudent to do so to permit inspection.

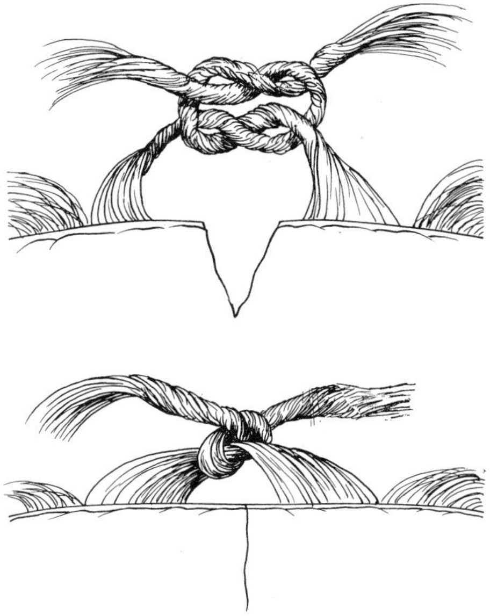

Aftercare
Suture removal

The earlier sutures are removed the less the likelihood of persistent puncture marks but the greater the risk of dehiscence. As a very approximate guide, sutures on the face should be removed after 4–5 days, on the trunk, thighs, and upper arms after 7–8 days, and on the hands and feet after 10–12 days. Wounds where the epidermis is thick and fibrous, particularly in the vicinity of joints and movement, will take longer to heal effectively then where the epidermis is thin with a good blood supply and little movement.

Analgesia

The effect of local anaesthetics used for minor surgery will rarely persist for more than an hour or

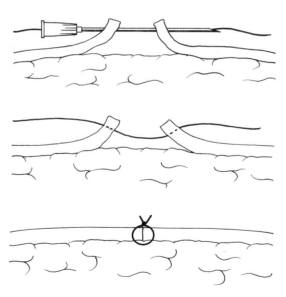

Fig. 5.14. Emergency suturing: the scalp.

Fig. 5.15. Emergency suturing: i.v. needle method.

so and will be wearing off by the time the patient gets home. Advice is therefore appropriate how the inevitable post-operative discomfort can be alleviated. The following suggestions may be helpful:

(1) rest the injured part—an ancient and effective maxim!;

(2) where a wound on a limb is involved, elevation of a leg or putting an arm in a high sling reduces oedema and vascular congestion and, thus, discomfort;

(3) when digits are involved, immobilization can be achieved by buddy strapping or the provision of a plaster of Paris cap;

(4) over-the-counter medication such as aspirin, paracetamol, or ibuprofen (Nurofen) usually affords sufficient relief until discomfort subsides.

Follow-up

Follow-up of cases treated by minor operation in general practice is important for a number of reasons:

(1) to assess the success of the procedure;

(2) to detect and manage actual or incipient complications;

(3) to check on histological reports and arrange a further opinion or treatment if indicated;

(4) to ensure that notes are complete for medico-legal reasons;

(5) to ensure that the appropriate claims for payment have been made;

(6) to complete statistical entries for the practice annual report and as an audit exercise;

(7) to confirm patient satisfaction.

Complications of minor surgery

Early

Syncope

Vasovagal attacks may occur in susceptible subjects of any age and either sex at any point during minor surgical procedures. The situation may be avoided both by effective pre-surgery counselling and by ensuring that the patient is recumbent during the operation. If such attacks do occur (pallor, bradycardia, sweating, loss of consciousness, jactitation) the procedure should be halted, the table tilted into the head-down position, and an airway inserted if necessary (see resuscitation equipment). Recovery usually occurs in a few minutes and the operation should be completed as expeditiously as possible. If bradycardia persists, administer atropine sulphate 600 µg intramuscularly or intraveneously by incremental doses of 100 µg until recovery occurs.

Haemorrhage

Control of bleeding has been discussed above. It is of vital importance for good results that haemostasis is achieved before sutures are inserted.

Haematoma

If a haematoma is seen to be forming as dressings are being applied, the wound must be taken down again and effective haemostatic control ensured before resuturing.

Pain

See suggestions above regarding management of pain.

Late

Infection

Infection developing in the post-operative period will be characterized by pain, inflammation, or purulent discharge. If cellulitis without abscess formation has occurred, prescribe a broad spectrum, penicillinase-resistant antibiotic, delay suture removal and observe daily until it has settled. If the infection should progress to abscess formation, however, remove sutures in the immediate locality and evacuate the pus. Take a swab for bacterial culture and sensitivity in case antibiotic therapy is indicated later. The wound will usually heal by second intention although excision of the resulitng scar may eventually be required.

Dehiscence

Wound dehiscence may occur as a result of infection, premature suture removal, poor opposition of incision edges, failure to obliterate subcutaneous cavities, haematoma formation, etc. It can best be prevented by scrupulous attention to operative technique. In the absence of ongoing infection, secondary suture after excision of the wound edges is appropriate.

Long term

Keloids

Keloid formation typically occurs where surgery is performed on the 'cape' area of the body (upper back, shoulders, and pectoral region). It is most prone to occur in patients of Afro-Carribean origin. Keloids sometimes respond to the application of steroid-impregnated adhesive strip (clobetasol proprionate—not available on FP10) or by multiple microinjections of triamcinolone acetonide (Adcortyl, Kenalog).

Contracture

Only likely to occur where incisions have been made in the vicinity of joints at right angles to the natural cutaneous flexure lines.

Loss of function

Possibly the result of inadvertent damage to deep structures such as tendons and nerves where procedures have been undertaken in the 'danger areas'.

Pigmentation

Pigmentation may occur as a result of the use of iron-containing haemostatic reagents (*quod vide*) or where blood has leaked from superficial vessels, for example, during sclerotherapy.

If complications occur, the reasons should be explained frankly to the patient and factually recorded in the notes together with any remedial measures that are taken.

References

Anon (1991). Local applications to wounds: II. Dressings for wounds and ulcers. *Drug and Therapeutics Bulletin*, **29**, 97–100.

Chew, C. (1991). Training for minor surgery in general practice during preregistration surgical posts. *British Medical Journal*, **302**, 1211–12.

Cox, N. H., Wagstaff, R., and Popple, A. W. (1992). Using clinicopathological analysis of general practitioner skin surgery to determine educational requirements and guidelines. *British Medical Journal*, **304**, 93–6.

Gibson, T. K. (1978). Langer (1819–1887) and his lines. *British Journal of Plastic Surgery*, **31**, 1–7.

Pringle, M., Hasler, J., and De Marco, P. (1991). Training for minor surgery in general practice during preregistration surgical posts. *British Medical Journal*, **302**, 830–2.

Further reading

Brown, J. S. (1992). *Minor surgery in general practice*, (2nd edn). RCGP, London.

Burge, S. and Rayment, R. (1986). *Simple skin surgery*. Blackwell Scientific Publications, Oxford.

Cracknell, I. and Mead, M. (1991). Introduction to minor surgery. *Update*, **421**, 247–58.

Fry, J., Higton, O., and Stephenson, J. (1990). *Colour atlas of minor surgery in general practice*. Kluwer Academic Publishers, London.

Milne, R. (1990). Minor surgery in general practice. *British Journal of General Practice*, **401**, 175–6.

Saleh, M. and Sodera, V. K. (1988). *Illustrated handbook of minor surgery and operative technique*. Heinemann Medical Books, London.

Snook, R. (1971). Minor surgery: skin closure. *Update Plus*, **11**, 287–95.

Stoddard, C. J. and Smith, J. A. R. (1985) *Complications of minor surgery*. Balliere Tindall, London.

Appendix A: Crease and wrinkle lines; Langer's lines

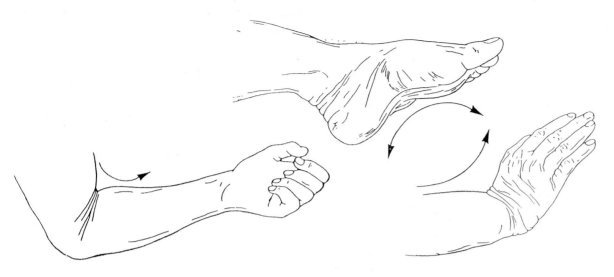

Crease and wrinkle lines

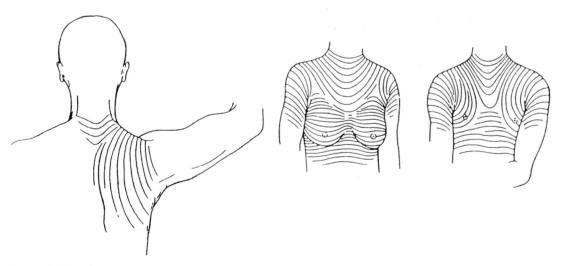

Langer's lines

Appendix B: Surgical sutures available on NHS prescription

Absorbable sutures
Sterile catgut chromic BP

Ethicon code no.	Metric gauge	Length	Needle
W480	2.0	75 cm	16 mm curved cutting
W548	2.0	75 cm	16 mm curved round bodied
W565	3.5	75 cm (extra chromic)	25 mm tapercut half-circle heavy
W488	3.5	75 cm	35 mm tapercut half-circle
W492	3.5	75 cm	45 mm tapercut half-circle heavy

Non-absorbable sutures
Sterile polymide 6 suture, monofilament BP

Ethicon code no.	Metric gauge	Length	Needle
W506	0.7	35 cm (black)	16 mm curved cutting
W507	0.7	45 cm (black)	15 mm slim blade curved cutting
W319	1.5	45 cm (blue)	19 cm curved reverse cutting
W539	1.5	45 cm (blue)	25 mm slim blade curved cutting
W320	2.0	45 cm (blue)	26 mm curved reverse

Sterile polyamide 66 suture, braided BP

Ethicon code no.	Metric gauge	Length	Needle
W5414	3.5	1 m (black)	50 mm tapercut half-circle heavy

Sterile braided silk suture BP

Ethicon code no.	Metric gauge	Length	Needle
W501	1.5	75 cm (black)	16 mm curved cutting
W533	2.0	45 cm (black)	25 mm super cutting curved
W321	3.0	45 cm (black)	26 mm curved reverse cutting
W667	3.0	75 cm (black)	35 mm curved reverse cutting

Skin closure strips, sterile (Steri-strip)

3 M code no.		
GP 41	6 mm × 75 mm	Three strips per envelope

Note: these items are specifically for personal administration by the prescriber.

Appendix C: Sterile dressing packs available on NHS prescription

These packs contain a selection of sterile dressings required in special nursing procedures (usually for post-operative re-dressing of wounds) when performed in the home. Prescribers have been advised to order this dressing only for an individual patient for whom such a sterile dressing operation is essential and to restrict their orders to the number of packs considered to be required for that patient. The exact number of packs ordered by the prescriber to be dispensed. A pack is to be used for each sterile dressing operation.

Sterile dressing pack
Specification 10
Sterile pack containing:
gauze and cotton tissue pad (8.5 cm × 20 cm),
gauze swabs 12 ply (4 × 10 cm × 10 cm),
absorbent cotton balls, large (4 × 0.9 g approximately),
absorbent paper towel (45 cm × 50 cm),
water repellent inner wrapper opens out as a sterile working field (50 cm × 50 cm).
To be supplied in the individual pack, sealed and sterilized as received from the manufacturer or wholesaler.

Sterile dressing pack with non-woven pads (Patient Ready)
Specification 35
Sterile pack containing:
non-woven fabric covered dressing pad (Surgipad) (10 cm × 20 cm),
non-woven fabric swabs (Topper 8) (4 × 10 cm × 10 cm),
absorbent cotton wool balls (4 × 0.8 g approximately),
absorbent paper towel (45 cm × 51 cm),
water repellent inner wrapper opens out as a sterile working field (50 cm × 50 cm).

Sterile knitted viscose dressing
Knitted viscose primary dressing BP. To be supplied in the individual pack sealed and sterilized as received from the manufacturer or wholesaler.
N-A dressing (9.5 cm × 9.5 cm)
Tricotex (9.5 cm × 9.5 cm).

6 Administration, records, and claims

Regulations

The regulations concerning the provision of minor surgery services by family practitioners and the utilization of such services by NHS patients are laid down in the *General medical services regulations* (NHS 1992), Paragraphs 32 and 33. This document covers applications by doctors to join the Family Health Service Authority (FHSA) Minor Surgery List, the required accreditation, appeals procedure, approval of premises (although criteria are not specified), eligibility of patients for the service, the list of approved procedures qualifying for payment (Schedule 6), and so on. The regulations and fee-claim procedures are also summarized in the NHS General Medical Services (1990) *Statement of fees and allowances* (the Red Book) Paragraphs 42.1–42.7 and Paragraph 42 Schedule 1 and are reproduced here in Appendix A and B and the extended list of procedures for fund-holding practices is reproduced in Appendix C. Appendix D summarizes the requirements for fund-holding practices to ensure quality control and competence.

The minor surgery list
Accreditation

Doctors wishing to claim payment for minor surgery sessions under the above NHS regulations must be included in the Minor Surgery List of a Family Health Service Authority and evidence of satisfactory training and experience will be required. Applicants should be able to show that they have a relevent postgraduate qualification in surgery or have undertaken an appropriate course of training or have had regular minor surgery experience during the 5 years prior to the application. In the latter respect, the production of a practice minor operations register would be appropriate evidence. For doctors qualified for general practice for less than 5 years, evidence of recent hospital experience during a vocational training course in a casualty or dermatology department would also be appropriate but, as Pringle *et al.* (1991) and Chew (1991), have pointed out, doubt has recently been cast on the adequacy of teaching of minor surgery during general house surgeon appointments in the pre-registration year. Doctors who do not fulfil the required criteria *ab initio* may achieve accreditation by attendance at a recognized theoretical course on minor surgery lasting at least 1 day (6 h) together with evidence of practical experience as recommended by their Regional General Practice Education Committee. Guidelines on training and the facilities required for minor surgery have been issued to Local Medical Committees, RCGP faculties, and Regional Advisors in General Practice (DHSS 1991) whence further advice may be obtained. According to the regulations, doctors providing minor surgery services are expected to be competent in performing all the procedures listed in the schedule although, in some circumstances, injection of varicose veins and haemorrhoids may be excluded.

Eligible patients

According to the *General medical service regulations* (NHS 1992), Paragraph 33, a doctor who is on the FHSA Minor Surgery list may provide services

(1) for any patient who is on his/her own NHS list;

(2) for any patient who is on the list of one of his or her partners;

(3) for any patient who is on the list of a doctor with whom he/she works in a group practice association (see *General medical services regulations* (NHS 1992), part I, 2.(1)).

When a doctor undertakes a minor surgical procedure for a patient who is not on his/her own list, he/she should inform the patient's own doctor in writing of the nature and outcome of the operation.

Organizing sessions

The NHS *Statement of fees and allowances*, Paragraph 42.2, (NHS General Medical Services 1990) defines a session as a total of five approved procedures performed by an individual practitioner. The procedures may, however, be performed either at a single clinic or on separate occasions and the significance of this, relating to the submission of claims for payment for minor surgery is considered below. Thus, although minor operations can be performed on an *ad hoc* basis (and, indeed, some, such as the removal of foreign bodies or the incision of acute abscesses, must be undertaken without delay), it is likely to prove more convenient for both doctors and practice nursing staff to set aside protected time, say, once a week, for a minor operating session. The time required for specific procedures can only be determined by experience. However, relevant factors include not only the time necessary for the operation itself (for example, injection of veins and excision procedures will perhaps require twice the time needed for cautery or steroid injections) but also the 'turn-around time' between patients. This means the time needed for setting up trolleys, preparing the patient, recovery after the procedure, stripping trolleys and clearing away equipment, resterilization of instruments, and

Table 6.1.

Long procedures	Short procedures
Injections	
Injection of varicose veins	Intra-articular injections
Injection of haemorrhoids	Peri-articular injections
	Soft tissue injections
Aspirations	
Hydrocele	Cyst in breast
	Cyst of epididymis
	Joints, bursae, and ganglions
Incisions	
Paronychia	Peri-anal abscess
Terminal pulp infection	Peri-anal haematoma
Meibomian cyst evacuation	Other superficial abscesses
Excisions	
Sebaceous cyst	Punch and shave biopsy
Lipoma	Papillomata
Ingrowing toenail	Toenail avulsion
Zadik procedure	
Subungual exostosis	
Cautery and cryotherapy	
Unless multiple lesions are being treated at one session, these will almost always fall into the 'short' category	
Other procedures	
Removal of foreign bodies will almost always be emergency rather than elective procedures. Other eligible operations will usually not be time-consuming	

disinfection of work surfaces, not to mention clerical procedures such as the completion of records. As a rough guide, longer operations will require approximately 30 min each whereas short procedures can be completed in perhaps 15 min. Table 6.1 offers an approximate classification.

Records
Minor operations register
A lasting record of minor operations within the practice is important for audit and fiscal, as well as for medico-legal, reasons. Minimal data should be

kept in a dedicated register retained in the treatment area which should include

(1) date and time of operation;
(2) patient identification, for example, name, sex, and date of birth;
(3) surgeon's name;
(4) name of assistant or nurse in attendance;
(5) nature of the procedure completed;
(6) type of anaesthesia/analgesia used;
(7) tissue sent for histology (if any);
(8) notes, for example, complications, variation from routine methods, etc.

A specimen page is shown in Appendix E and it should be the responsibility of the treatment room nurse to confirm that all procedures, whether or not included in the schedule approved for payment, are recorded therein.

Clinical notes
As with any other doctor–patient contact, a note should always be made in the patient's NHS records regarding minor surgical procedures performed, follow-up consultations, complications, etc. This is the only record that will follow the patient to subsequent medical attendants and, thus, provide a definitive history of the event.

Doctor's work sheet
Although a record of minor operations is retained in the treatment area (see above), in a multi partner practice it may not be easy for clerical staff compiling claims for payment (see below) to classify procedures correctly for each doctor. Moreover, some simple procedures, for example, soft tissue injections or aspiration of a bursa, may have been done in the consulting room and entry into the Minor Operations Register subsequently

overlooked. The submission of claims can be considerably simplified if each doctor in the group keeps a personal work sheet for minor surgery (for example, Appendix F) wherein he/she can identify the patient and classify the procedure appropriately at the time of operation. At the end of each quarter, the clerk simply has to total the procedures in each category column and enter the results against the doctor's name on Claim Form FP/MS (Rev) (Appendix G). Furthermore, should the FHSA question the authenticity of a practitioner's claim (NHS *Statement of fees and allowances* (the Red Book), Paragraph 42.7 (NHS General Medical Services 1990)), detailed information regarding the procedures undertaken by that particular doctor during that quarter will be readily to hand.

Submitting claims for fees
Restrictions†
Numbers
Individual practitioners may claim for not more than three sessions (15 approved procedures) in a single quarter (NHS *Statement of fees and allowances* (the Red Book) Paragraph 42.1 (NHS General Medical Services 1990)). However, where a doctor is a member of a partnership or group practice, he or she may claim a higher number of payments, provided that the total number of sessional payments made to the partnership or group in that quarter does not exceed three times the total number of practitioners in the group, whether or not they are on the Minor Surgery List of the FHSA. For example, a partnership of five doctors could claim up to 15 sessions, a total of 75 procedures, each quarter irrespective of how many doctors were

For fund-holding practices, regulations regarding numbers and procedures were extended in 1993 (see Appendix C).

on the Minor Surgery List or how many each performed individually.

Qualifying procedures
In spite of the list of procedures qualifying for payment detailed in Schedule 1 of the NHS *Statement of fees and allowances*, Paragraph 42 (NHS General Medical Services 1990), doubt is sometimes expressed by FHSAs concerning the eligibility of certain operations. For example, whilst the injection of steroid solutions into tennis or golfer's elbow may legitimately be regarded as peri-articular, the injection of policeman's heel may not. Similarly, whilst injection of varicose veins is allowable, injection of teleangiectasia or spider naevi for cosmetic purposes may not be so. Whilst the authors of this handbook have taken pains to illustrate procedures that, in their understanding, qualify for payment, there may still be anomalies and, if there is doubt, readers are advised to take advice from the appointed Medical Advisors at their FHSAs.

Claims procedure
Claims for fees for minor surgery must be submitted to FHSAs by practices for individual doctors at the end of each quarter on form FP/MS (Rev) which is reproduced in Appendix F. The total number of each type of procedure undertaken by each doctor must be entered even if the maximum for payment purposes has been exceeded (see Appendix F, Note 3). The excess may then be carried forward to the next quarter (NHS *Statement of fees and allowances*, Paragraph 42.3 (NHS General Medical Services 1990)) and will, in any event, provide the FHSA with a measure of the prevalence of 'unfunded' procedures.

References
Chew, C. (1991). Training for minor surgery in general practice during preregistration surgical posts. *British Medical Journal*, **302**, 1211–12.

Department of Health and Social Security (1991). *Minor surgery in general practice.* Guidelines by the General Medical Services Committee and the Royal College of General Practitioners in collaboration with the Royal College of Surgeons of England and the Royal College of Surgeons of Edinburgh and the Joint Committee on Postgraduate Training for General Practice. DHSS, London.

National Health Service (1992). *General medical services regulations.* HMSO, London.

National Health Service General Medical Services (1990). *Statement of fees and allowances payable to general medical practitioners in England and Wales from 1 April, 1990.* Department of Health Welsh Office, London.

Pringle, M., Hasler, J., and De Marco, P. (1991). Training for minor surgery in general practice during preregistration surgical posts. *British Medical Journal*, **302**, 830–2.

Further reading
National Health Service Management Executive. Health Service Guidelines HSG(93)14. *GP fund-holding practices: the provision of secondary care.* DoH, London.

Appendix A: NHS statement of fees and allowances regulations

Minor surgery

Eligibility

42.1 The fee in Paragraph 1 Schedule 1 for minor surgery will be payable to a practitioner on the FHSA's Minor Surgery List who provides a minor surgery session as set out below for patients on his or her personal list or the personal list of his or her partner or another member of the group. A practitioner will be eligible for no more than three such payments in respect of any quarter. Where a practitioner is a member of a partnership or group he or she may claim a higher number of payments, provided that the total number of payments paid to the partnership or group in respect of any one quarter shall not exceed three times the number of the partners or members of the group on the Medical List of the FHSA on the first day of the quarter.

Definition of a session

42.2 A session will consist of five surgical procedures performed by an individual practitioner. Practitioners may conduct a session either by performing the procedures in a single clinic or on separate occasions.

42.3 A practitioner on the Minor Surgery List may carry forward up to four procedures into the following quarter provided the procedures were performed within the three quarters preceding it.

42.4 Procedures will count towards a session provided:

(1) they are included in the list in Schedule 1;
(2) they are performed by a practitioner on the FHSA's Minor Surgery List;
(3) any other person assisting in the surgery (but not performing it) is suitably trained and/or experienced for the tasks they are required to undertake or if undergoing training is directly supervised by a suitably trained and/or experienced person.

Minor surgery list

42.5 A practitioner should apply to the FHSA for inclusion on the Minor Surgery List. The criteria which the FHSA will take into account in determining these applications are contained in Regulation 32.

Claims

42.6 Claims should be made on form FP/MS obtainable from the FHSA. This form will record details of the practitioner who performs the surgery and the date and type (using the categories in Schedule 1) of procedure carried out.

42.7 A practitioner wishing to claim a sessional fee should submit to the FHSA the appropriate form referred to in Paragraph 42.6 above. A practitioner should submit claim forms for complete sessions (that is, for five procedures) only. Where procedures are carried forward under Paragraph 42.3, the practitioner is responsible for maintaining a record containing information relating to the procedure until a claim which includes that procedure is made. Only one practitioner may claim payment in respect of any one procedure. The authenticity of claims will be the subject of checks by the FHSA with patients. Practitioners should therefore keep a record of the names of the patients involved.

**Appendix B: schedule of minor surgical procedures
for which payment may be made**

Paragraph 42 Schedule 1: **minor surgical procedures
for which payment may be made**
The following procedures will count towards
eligibility for payment of a fee.

1. Injections: intra-articular, peri-articular,
   varicose veins, and haemorrhoids.
2. Aspirations: joints, cysts, bursae, and
   hydrocele.
3. Incisions: abscesses, cysts, and thrombosed
   piles.
4. Excisions: sebaceous cysts, lipoma, skin
   lesions for histology, intradermal naevi,
   papilloma, dermatofibroma, and similar
   conditions, warts, and removal of toenails
   (partial and complete).
5. Curette, cautery, and cryocautery: warts and
   verrucae and other skin lesions, for example,
   molluscum contagiosum.
6. Other: removal of foreign bodies and nasal
   cautery.

Appendix C: Services in respect of which a member of a fund-holding practice may receive payment; HSG(93)14 Annex B

Pathology
Blood counts.
Tests for liver function and electrolytes.

Ophthalmology
Chalazion operation.
Operations for obstruction of the nasolacrimal duct.

ENT
Puncture of maxillary antrum with washout.
Pharyngoscopy.
Laryngoscopy.

General surgery
Endoscopy (upper gastrointestinal tract).
Sigmoidoscopy.
Ligation of varicose veins (below knee).

Genito-urinary surgery
Diagnostic flexible cystoscopy.
Vasectomy.

Gynaecology
Colposcopy.
Marsupialization of Bartholin's cyst.

Orthopaedics
Excision of ganglion.
Carpal tunnel release.

Other
Diagnostic ultrasound (not obstetric).

**Appendix D: Health Service Guidelines HSG(93)14
Annex C**

Quality and competence

In considering whether applicants have sufficient
competence to carry out the procedures for which
the application is made, regions should have regard
to the following:

(1) Training, qualifications, continuing
experience, and education (for example,
including case mix and caseload) of the GP
in the particular procedures, including
appropriate anaesthesia.

(2) Suitability of premises and equipment.

(3) Adequacy of back-up facilities.

(4) Training and experience of support staff.

(5) Arrangements to assess the quality of
treatment provided.

(6) Post-operative care and discharge
arrangements.

(7) Audit arrangements.

Appendix E: minor operations register (specimen page)

MINOR OPERATIONS REGISTER

Date	Patient's name	Sex	DoB	Procedure	Surgeon	Nurse	Anaesthetic	Histology?	Notes

50

Appendix F: Doctor's personal minor surgery work sheet

MINOR SURGERY WORKSHEET

Doctor's name: . . . .

Quarter commencing (please circle):

Jan.   Apr.   Jul.   Oct.   19 . . . .

Tick one

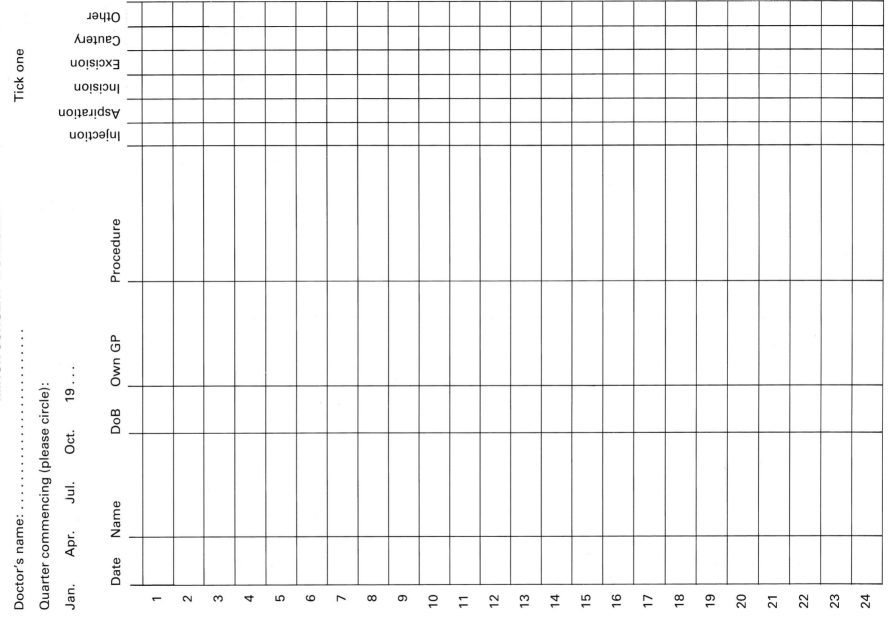

	Date	Name	DoB	Own GP	Procedure	Injection	Aspiration	Incision	Excision	Cautery	Other
1											
2											
3											
4											
5											
6											
7											
8											
9											
10											
11											
12											
13											
14											
15											
16											
17											
18											
19											
20											
21											
22											
23											
24											

Appendix G: Minor surgery fee claim form FP/MS (Rev)

Minor Surgery Fee Claim

Fill in one of these forms for *all* minor surgery procedures carried out in the practice during a quarter. (For more information, see SFA Paragraph 42)

Details of claiming practice

Doctor(s) _____

Address _____

Period of claim

Quarter ending

☐ 30 June

☐ 30 September

☐ 31 December

☐ 31 March

Year of claim _____

Total number of procedures _____ (See note 3)

(Please give below details of each category of procedure, see notes on reverse)

Name of doctor who carried out procedure(s) (see note 1)	No/Type of procedure (See SFA Paragraph 42, Schedule 1 and note 2)						
	Injection	Aspiration	Incision	Excision	Cauterization	Others	Total
Total							

Declaration

I certify that the information shown on this form is correct.

I claim payment in accordance with the Statement of Fees and Allowances.

Senior partners signature _____

Date _____

Notes

1. Please enter doctors name in block capitals for clarity.

2. Enter in each box, the number of procedures undertaken by each doctor in each category, then total down and across.

3. Enter total number of procedures carried out in the practice by eligible doctors in the space provided. (Please enter *all* procedures carried out in the quarter even if you exceed your maximum for payment purposes as this provides the FHSA with an indication of 'unfunded' procedures.

4. The FHSA reserves the right to check the authenticity of claims and it is therefore recommended that adequate records are kept in the surgery. The use of a minor surgery book will assist you in completing this quarterly claim form. The record should include patient details, date of surgery, type of procedure, anaesthetic used, and staff involved.

5. See Paragraph 42.3 of the SFA for criteria on carry forward of procedures.

7 Procedures appropriate to the new contract

Injections: Intra-articular and peri-articular

Introduction

It is now more than 40 years since the dramatic anti-inflammatory effect of locally injected steroids was described by Hollander and McCarty and this form of therapy has subsequently transformed the management of many musculo-skeletal and rheumatological conditions. Although pure hydrocortisone is too soluble and thus, diffuses quickly from the injection site, isomers prepared in a microcrystalline form provide a stable suspension that, when deposited at the site of an inflammatory lesion, will persist and exert a continuing anti-inflammatory effect for several weeks. Over the years, synthetic analogues have been developed and Table 7.1 lists the preparations presently available in the United Kingdom.

Principles and technique

Success with topical injection of inflammatory lesions will only develop with practice and experience but is, overall, a relatively safe method of treatment provided that the basic principles, summarized here, are observed.

1. A firm diagnosis of the pathological nature of the lesion must first be established.

Table 7.1. Corticosteroid preparations available for local injection

Generic name	Proprietary name	Manufacturer	Availability
Shorter duration			
Hydrocortisone acetate	Hydrocortistab	Boots	25 mg per ml 1 ml ampoule
Prednisolone acetate	Deltastab	Boots	25 mg per ml 1 ml ampoule
Longer duration			
Methylprednisolone acetate	Depo-Medrone	Upjohn	40 mg per ml 1, 2, and 3 ml vial
Methylprednisolone acetate, lignocaine 1 per cent	Depo-Medrone with Lidocaine	Upjohn	40 mg per ml 1 and 2 ml vial
Triamcinolone acetonide	Adcortyl	Squibb	10 mg per ml 1 ml ampoule 5 ml vial
Triamcinolone acetonide	Kenalog	Squibb	40 mg per ml 1 ml vial

2. The physician must be conversant with the regional anatomy of the area to be injected and, in particular, its relationship to other important structures.
3. The injection site should be carefully marked before proceeding.
4. Scrupulous attention must be paid to aseptic technique.
5. The nature and duration of effect and dose of the steroid preparation selected should be appropriate to the condition under treatment.
6. Because of the dystrophic effect of steroids, they should, with certain exceptions (for example, keloids, fibrositis nodules) be injected only into potential tissue spaces such as the synovial cavities of joints and bursae. Injection into the substance of tendons and nerves must be rigorously avoided.
7. Lack of resistance when injecting often gives confirmation of correct placement.
8. The use of a local anaesthetic solution (for example, lignocaine 1 per cent) mixed with the steroid will not only make the procedure less painful for the patient but will also, especially in the case of muscular and ligamentous lesions, by the immediate relief of pain, confirm that the steroid has been infiltrated correctly.

The procedures illustrated in this section do not claim to be exhaustive; indeed, one procedure in particular, injection of the hip joint, has purposely been omitted, it being the opinion of the author that expertise in this instance is more appropriate to the specialist rheumatologist than to the general practitioner.

Further reading

Dixon, A. St J. and Graber, J. (1981). *Local injection therapy in rheumatic diseases*. Monograph Series No. 4, Eular Publishers, Basle.

Hollander, J. L., Jessar, R. A., and Brown, E. M. (1961). Intra-synovial corticosteroid therapy: a decade of use. *Bulletin on Rheumatic Diseases*, **11**, 279–40.

Nichol, F. (1992). Injection of the painful shoulder. *Update*, **44**, 39–44.

Silver, T. (1986). Injecting soft tissue lesions with confidence: the shoulder. *Modern Medicine*, **86**, 17–24.

The two conditions affecting the shoulder joint most commonly encountered in general practice are rotator cuff syndrome (supraspinatus tendonitis) and adhesive capsulitis (frozen shoulder). Both respond well to injection with steroid substances but, since they involve different synovial cavities of the joint, the injection sites are not the same and the differential diagnosis is therefore important.

Equipment Depo-Medrone with Lidocaine (1 ml/40 mg)

2 ml syringe

Mediswab

skin pencil   blue gauge needle

Anatomy

coracoacromial ligament
acromioclavicular joint
supraspinatus tendon
acromion
clavicle
subacromial bursa
humeral head
joint capsule
coracoid process
deltoid
scapula

1. The rotator cuff syndrome is characterised by a painful arc of movement of the abducted arm, 45 degrees above and below the horizontal plane.

2. Palpate the depression between the acromion and the head of the humerus and mark with the skin pencil.

clavicle
acromion
humeral head

3. Insert the needle about 15 mm up, under the acromion at an angle of 10 degrees to the horizontal. Inject 0.5 to 1.0 ml Depo-Medrone depending on the size of the patient. The injection should be painless and, if correctly positioned, the lignocaine in it should promptly relieve the painful arc syndrome.

4. Test for adhesive capsulitis by asking the patient to flex the forearm to 90 degrees and hold the elbow against the patient's side. Medial and lateral rotation of the forearm will be limited and painful.

5. Palpate the coracoid process and the head of the humerus. Mark the depression between them immediately lateral to the coracoid.

6. With the needle almost in the sagittal plane, enter the glenoid cavity and inject 1.0 ml Depo-Medrone. There should be no resistance to injection of the solution.

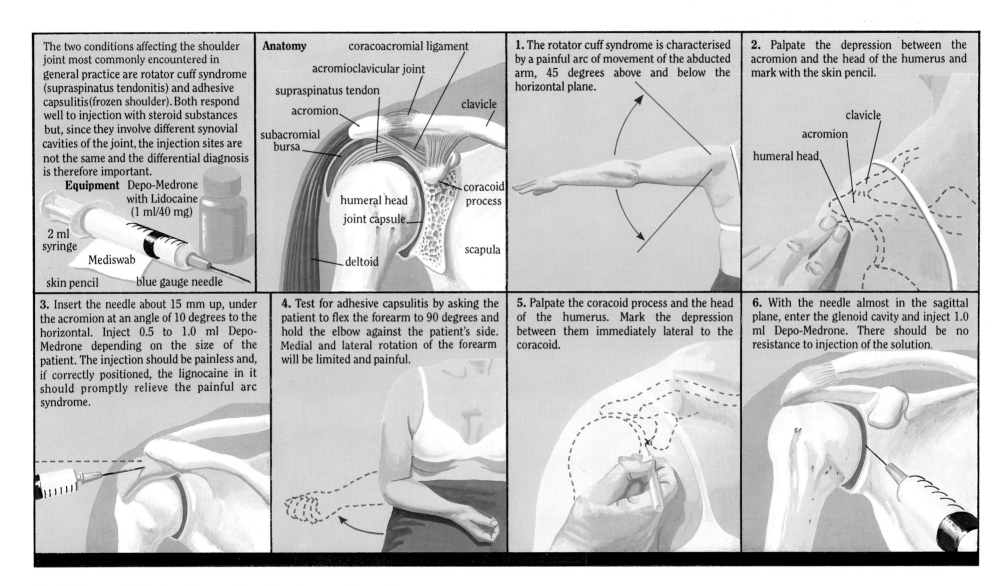

Fig. 7.1. Intra-articular: shoulder—rotator cuff syndrome and capsulitis.

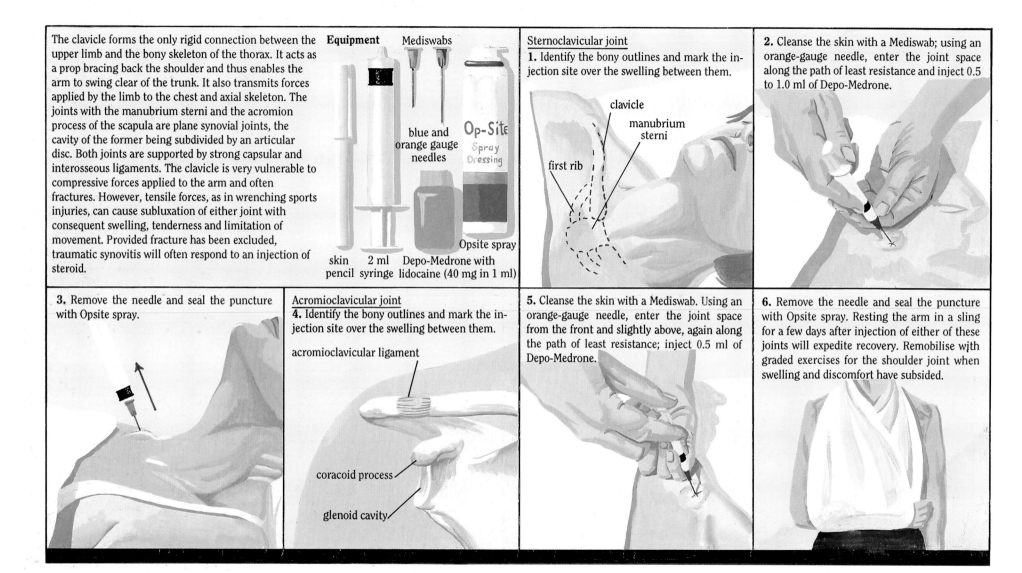

The clavicle forms the only rigid connection between the upper limb and the bony skeleton of the thorax. It acts as a prop bracing back the shoulder and thus enables the arm to swing clear of the trunk. It also transmits forces applied by the limb to the chest and axial skeleton. The joints with the manubrium sterni and the acromion process of the scapula are plane synovial joints, the cavity of the former being subdivided by an articular disc. Both joints are supported by strong capsular and interosseous ligaments. The clavicle is very vulnerable to compressive forces applied to the arm and often fractures. However, tensile forces, as in wrenching sports injuries, can cause subluxation of either joint with consequent swelling, tenderness and limitation of movement. Provided fracture has been excluded, traumatic synovitis will often respond to an injection of steroid.

Equipment   Mediswabs

blue and orange gauge needles

Op-Site Spray Dressing

Opsite spray

skin pencil   2 ml syringe   Depo-Medrone with lidocaine (40 mg in 1 ml)

Sternoclavicular joint
1. Identify the bony outlines and mark the injection site over the swelling between them.

clavicle

manubrium sterni

first rib

2. Cleanse the skin with a Mediswab; using an orange-gauge needle, enter the joint space along the path of least resistance and inject 0.5 to 1.0 ml of Depo-Medrone.

3. Remove the needle and seal the puncture with Opsite spray.

Acromioclavicular joint
4. Identify the bony outlines and mark the injection site over the swelling between them.

acromioclavicular ligament

coracoid process

glenoid cavity

5. Cleanse the skin with a Mediswab. Using an orange-gauge needle, enter the joint space from the front and slightly above, again along the path of least resistance; inject 0.5 ml of Depo-Medrone.

6. Remove the needle and seal the puncture with Opsite spray. Resting the arm in a sling for a few days after injection of either of these joints will expedite recovery. Remobilise with graded exercises for the shoulder joint when swelling and discomfort have subsided.

Fig. 7.2. Intra-articular: sterno-clavicular and acromio-clavicular joints.

The small joints of the hand are prone to osteoarthritic degenerative change in the elderly with consequent deformity, pain and loss of function. Previous injury or rheumatoid arthritis are predisposing factors. Symptoms can often be ameliorated by injection of a long-acting steroid solution. The first carpo-metacarpal joint is commonly affected but the principles illustrated here can be applied to any small joint in the hand.

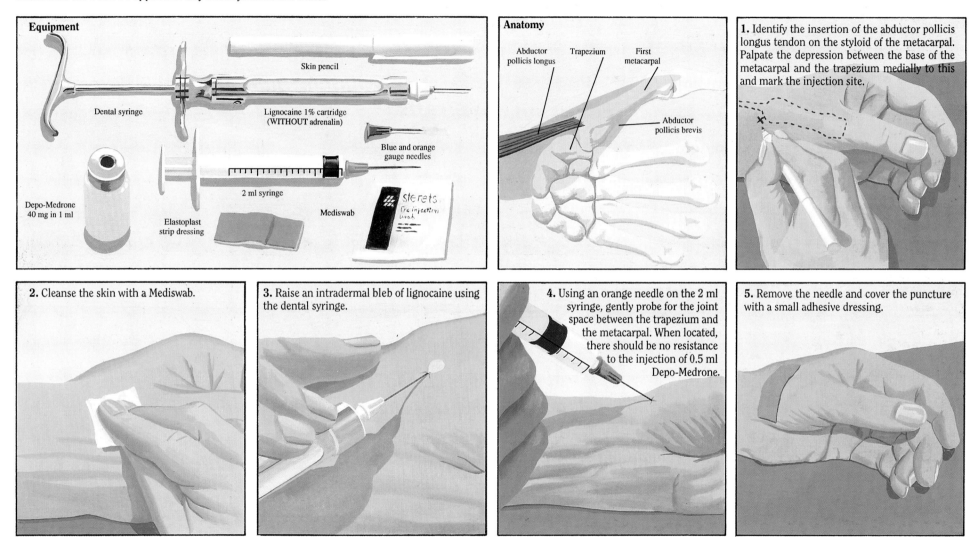

Fig. 7.3. Intra-articular: interphalangeal (I/P) and metacarpo-phalangeal (MC/P) joints.

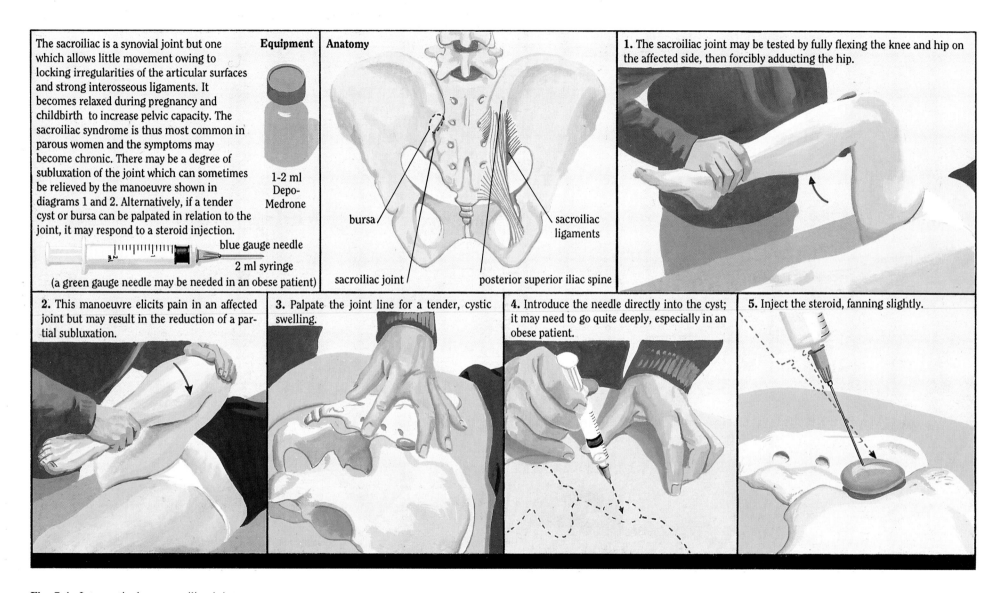

The sacroiliac is a synovial joint but one which allows little movement owing to locking irregularities of the articular surfaces and strong interosseous ligaments. It becomes relaxed during pregnancy and childbirth to increase pelvic capacity. The sacroiliac syndrome is thus most common in parous women and the symptoms may become chronic. There may be a degree of subluxation of the joint which can sometimes be relieved by the manoeuvre shown in diagrams 1 and 2. Alternatively, if a tender cyst or bursa can be palpated in relation to the joint, it may respond to a steroid injection.

Equipment

1-2 ml
Depo-
Medrone

blue gauge needle
2 ml syringe
(a green gauge needle may be needed in an obese patient)

Anatomy

bursa

sacroiliac joint

sacroiliac ligaments

posterior superior iliac spine

1. The sacroiliac joint may be tested by fully flexing the knee and hip on the affected side, then forcibly adducting the hip.

2. This manoeuvre elicits pain in an affected joint but may result in the reduction of a partial subluxation.

3. Palpate the joint line for a tender, cystic swelling.

4. Introduce the needle directly into the cyst; it may need to go quite deeply, especially in an obese patient.

5. Inject the steroid, fanning slightly.

Fig. 7.4. Intra-articular: sacro-iliac joint.

The supraspinatus muscle originates in the supraspinatus fossa of the scapula, its fibres converging under the acromion process to form a tendon which is inserted into the head of the humerus. Its prime function is to initiate and facilitate abduction of the arm at the shoulder joint. The tendon passes through the subacromial bursa and is frequently involved in the symptom complex known as painful arc syndrome. The patient is often middle-aged and an X-ray of the shoulder joint will sometimes show calcification in the tendon between the acromion and the humeral head. Supraspinatus tendonitis responds well to local steroid injection.

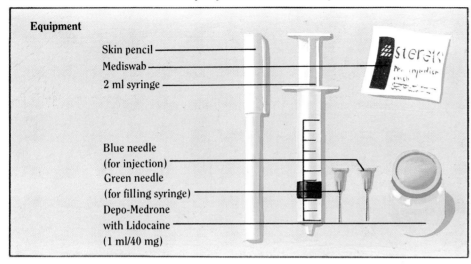

Equipment

Skin pencil

Mediswab

2 ml syringe

Blue needle
(for injection)

Green needle
(for filling syringe)

Depo-Medrone
with Lidocaine
(1 ml/40 mg)

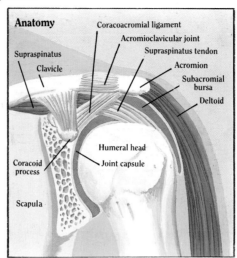

Anatomy

Coracoacromial ligament
Acromioclavicular joint
Supraspinatus tendon
Supraspinatus
Clavicle
Acromion
Subacromial bursa
Deltoid
Humeral head
Coracoid process
Joint capsule
Scapula

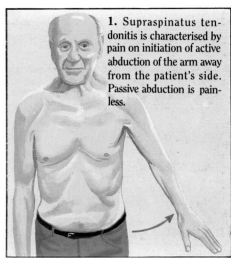

1. Supraspinatus tendonitis is characterised by pain on initiation of active abduction of the arm away from the patient's side. Passive abduction is painless.

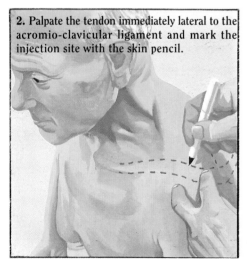

2. Palpate the tendon immediately lateral to the acromio-clavicular ligament and mark the injection site with the skin pencil.

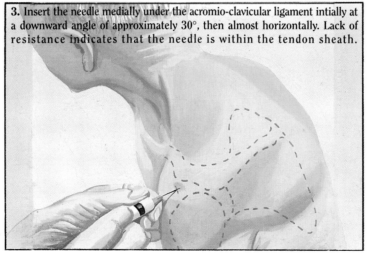

3. Insert the needle medially under the acromio-clavicular ligament intially at a downward angle of approximately 30°, then almost horizontally. Lack of resistance indicates that the needle is within the tendon sheath.

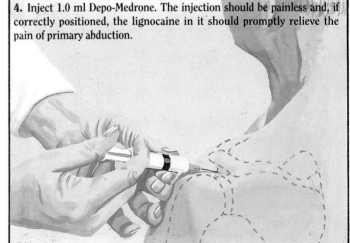

4. Inject 1.0 ml Depo-Medrone. The injection should be painless and, if correctly positioned, the lignocaine in it should promptly relieve the pain of primary abduction.

Fig. 7.5. Tendon sheath: supraspinatus tendonitis.

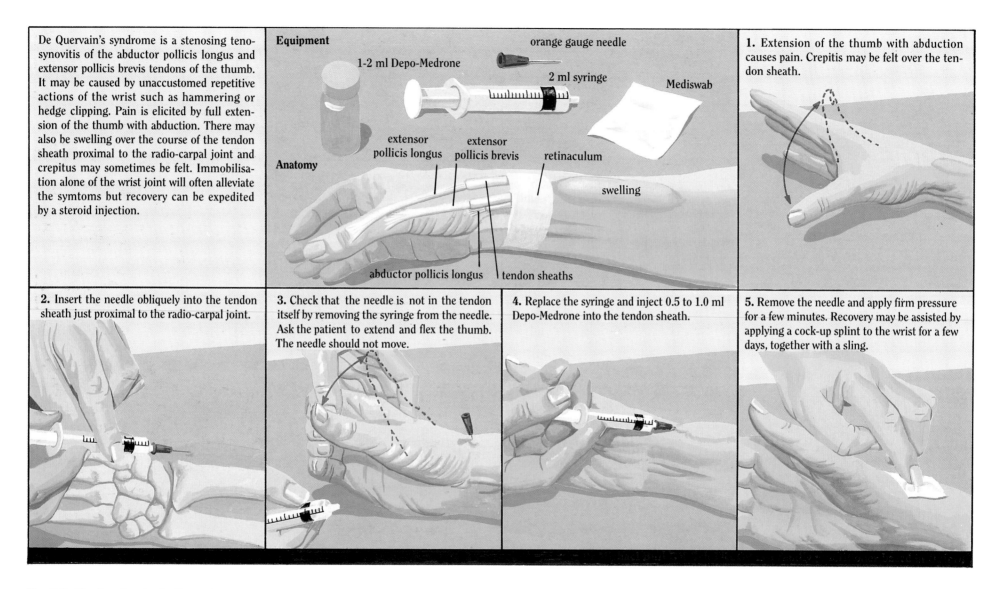

De Quervain's syndrome is a stenosing teno-synovitis of the abductor pollicis longus and extensor pollicis brevis tendons of the thumb. It may be caused by unaccustomed repetitive actions of the wrist such as hammering or hedge clipping. Pain is elicited by full extension of the thumb with abduction. There may also be swelling over the course of the tendon sheath proximal to the radio-carpal joint and crepitus may sometimes be felt. Immobilisation alone of the wrist joint will often alleviate the symtoms but recovery can be expedited by a steroid injection.

Equipment

orange gauge needle

1-2 ml Depo-Medrone

2 ml syringe

Mediswab

Anatomy

extensor pollicis longus

extensor pollicis brevis

retinaculum

swelling

abductor pollicis longus

tendon sheaths

1. Extension of the thumb with abduction causes pain. Crepitis may be felt over the tendon sheath.

2. Insert the needle obliquely into the tendon sheath just proximal to the radio-carpal joint.

3. Check that the needle is not in the tendon itself by removing the syringe from the needle. Ask the patient to extend and flex the thumb. The needle should not move.

4. Replace the syringe and inject 0.5 to 1.0 ml Depo-Medrone into the tendon sheath.

5. Remove the needle and apply firm pressure for a few minutes. Recovery may be assisted by applying a cock-up splint to the wrist for a few days, together with a sling.

Fig. 7.6. Tendon sheath: de Quervain's tendonitis.

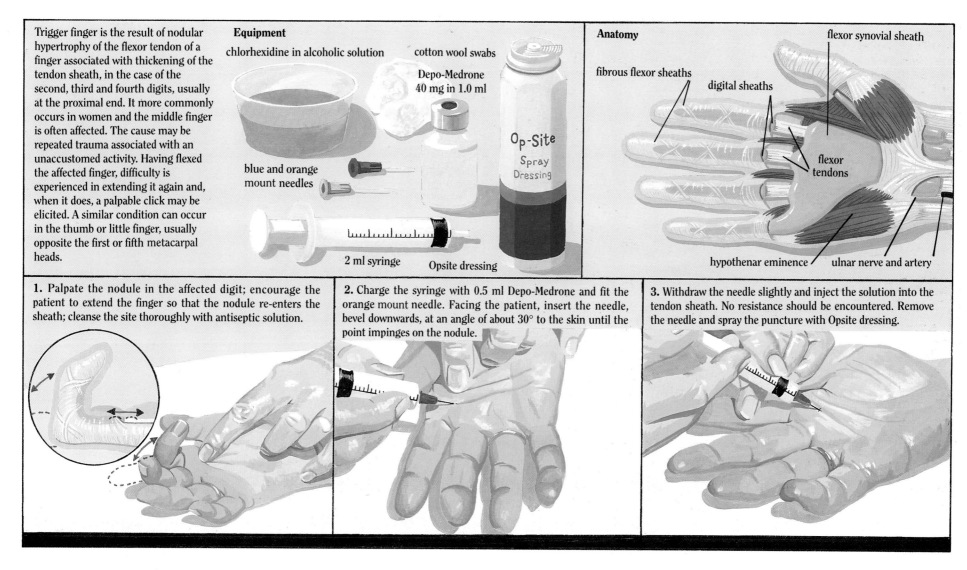

Trigger finger is the result of nodular hypertrophy of the flexor tendon of a finger associated with thickening of the tendon sheath, in the case of the second, third and fourth digits, usually at the proximal end. It more commonly occurs in women and the middle finger is often affected. The cause may be repeated trauma associated with an unaccustomed activity. Having flexed the affected finger, difficulty is experienced in extending it again and, when it does, a palpable click may be elicited. A similar condition can occur in the thumb or little finger, usually opposite the first or fifth metacarpal heads.

Equipment

chlorhexidine in alcoholic solution

cotton wool swabs

Depo-Medrone 40 mg in 1.0 ml

blue and orange mount needles

Op-Site Spray Dressing

2 ml syringe

Opsite dressing

Anatomy

fibrous flexor sheaths

digital sheaths

flexor synovial sheath

flexor tendons

hypothenar eminence

ulnar nerve and artery

1. Palpate the nodule in the affected digit; encourage the patient to extend the finger so that the nodule re-enters the sheath; cleanse the site thoroughly with antiseptic solution.

2. Charge the syringe with 0.5 ml Depo-Medrone and fit the orange mount needle. Facing the patient, insert the needle, bevel downwards, at an angle of about 30° to the skin until the point impinges on the nodule.

3. Withdraw the needle slightly and inject the solution into the tendon sheath. No resistance should be encountered. Remove the needle and spray the puncture with Opsite dressing.

Fig. 7.7. Tendon sheath: trigger finger/thumb.

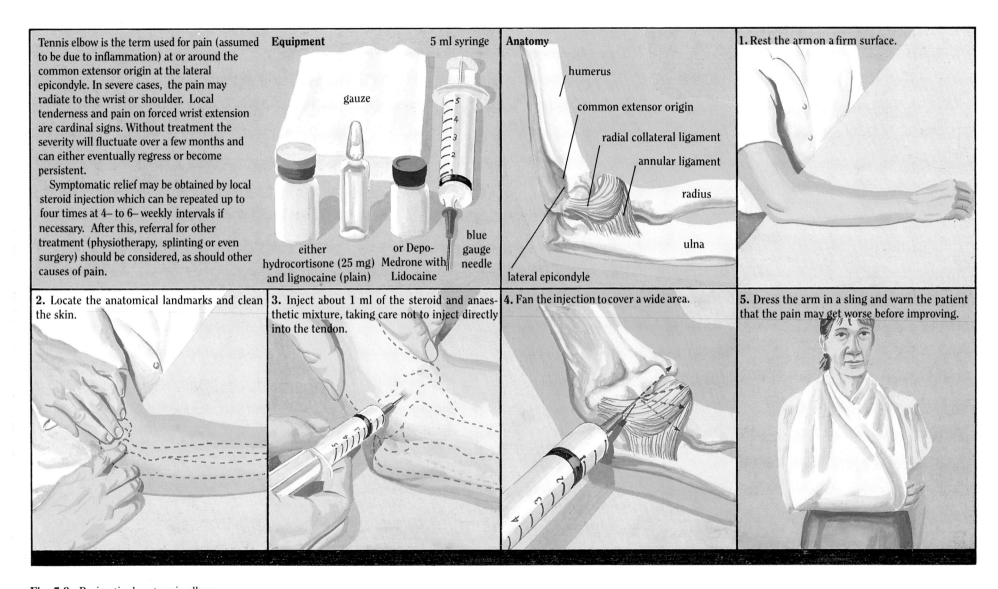

Tennis elbow is the term used for pain (assumed to be due to inflammation) at or around the common extensor origin at the lateral epicondyle. In severe cases, the pain may radiate to the wrist or shoulder. Local tenderness and pain on forced wrist extension are cardinal signs. Without treatment the severity will fluctuate over a few months and can either eventually regress or become persistent.

Symptomatic relief may be obtained by local steroid injection which can be repeated up to four times at 4– to 6– weekly intervals if necessary. After this, referral for other treatment (physiotherapy, splinting or even surgery) should be considered, as should other causes of pain.

Equipment   5 ml syringe

gauze

either hydrocortisone (25 mg) and lignocaine (plain)

or Depo-Medrone with Lidocaine

blue gauge needle

Anatomy

humerus

common extensor origin

radial collateral ligament

annular ligament

radius

ulna

lateral epicondyle

1. Rest the arm on a firm surface.

2. Locate the anatomical landmarks and clean the skin.

3. Inject about 1 ml of the steroid and anaesthetic mixture, taking care not to inject directly into the tendon.

4. Fan the injection to cover a wide area.

5. Dress the arm in a sling and warn the patient that the pain may get worse before improving.

Fig. 7.8. Peri-articular: tennis elbow.

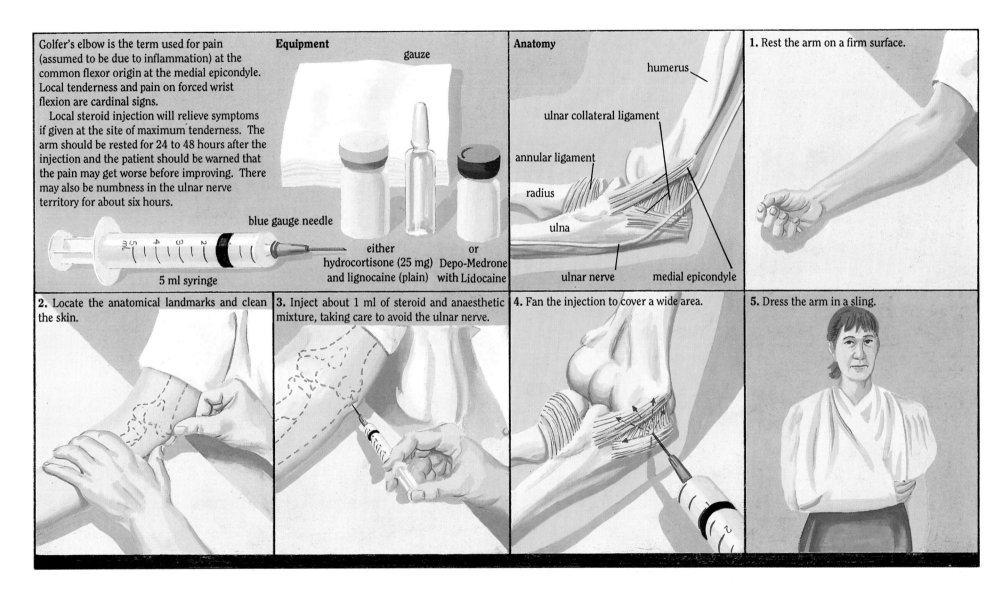

Golfer's elbow is the term used for pain (assumed to be due to inflammation) at the common flexor origin at the medial epicondyle. Local tenderness and pain on forced wrist flexion are cardinal signs.

Local steroid injection will relieve symptoms if given at the site of maximum tenderness. The arm should be rested for 24 to 48 hours after the injection and the patient should be warned that the pain may get worse before improving. There may also be numbness in the ulnar nerve territory for about six hours.

5 ml syringe

Equipment

gauze

blue gauge needle

either
hydrocortisone (25 mg) and lignocaine (plain)

or
Depo-Medrone with Lidocaine

Anatomy

humerus

ulnar collateral ligament

annular ligament

radius

ulna

ulnar nerve

medial epicondyle

1. Rest the arm on a firm surface.

2. Locate the anatomical landmarks and clean the skin.

3. Inject about 1 ml of steroid and anaesthetic mixture, taking care to avoid the ulnar nerve.

4. Fan the injection to cover a wide area.

5. Dress the arm in a sling.

Fig. 7.9. Peri-articular: golfer's elbow.

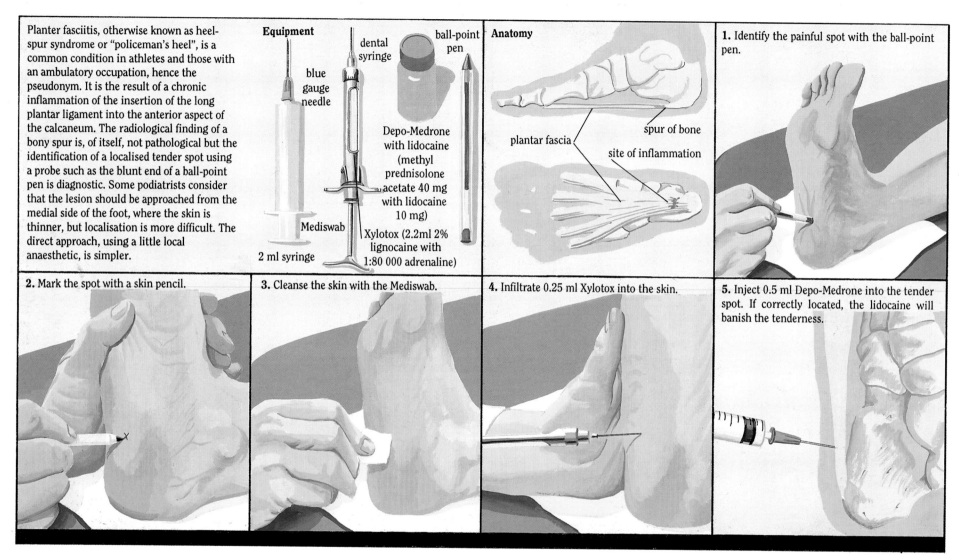

Planter fasciitis, otherwise known as heel-spur syndrome or "policeman's heel", is a common condition in athletes and those with an ambulatory occupation, hence the pseudonym. It is the result of a chronic inflammation of the insertion of the long plantar ligament into the anterior aspect of the calcaneum. The radiological finding of a bony spur is, of itself, not pathological but the identification of a localised tender spot using a probe such as the blunt end of a ball-point pen is diagnostic. Some podiatrists consider that the lesion should be approached from the medial side of the foot, where the skin is thinner, but localisation is more difficult. The direct approach, using a little local anaesthetic, is simpler.

Equipment

blue gauge needle

dental syringe

ball-point pen

Depo-Medrone with lidocaine (methyl prednisolone acetate 40 mg with lidocaine 10 mg)

Mediswab

Xylotox (2.2ml 2% lignocaine with 1:80 000 adrenaline)

2 ml syringe

Anatomy

plantar fascia

spur of bone

site of inflammation

1. Identify the painful spot with the ball-point pen.

2. Mark the spot with a skin pencil.

3. Cleanse the skin with the Mediswab.

4. Infiltrate 0.25 ml Xylotox into the skin.

5. Inject 0.5 ml Depo-Medrone into the tender spot. If correctly located, the lidocaine will banish the tenderness.

Fig. 7.10. Peri-articular: plantar fasciitis.

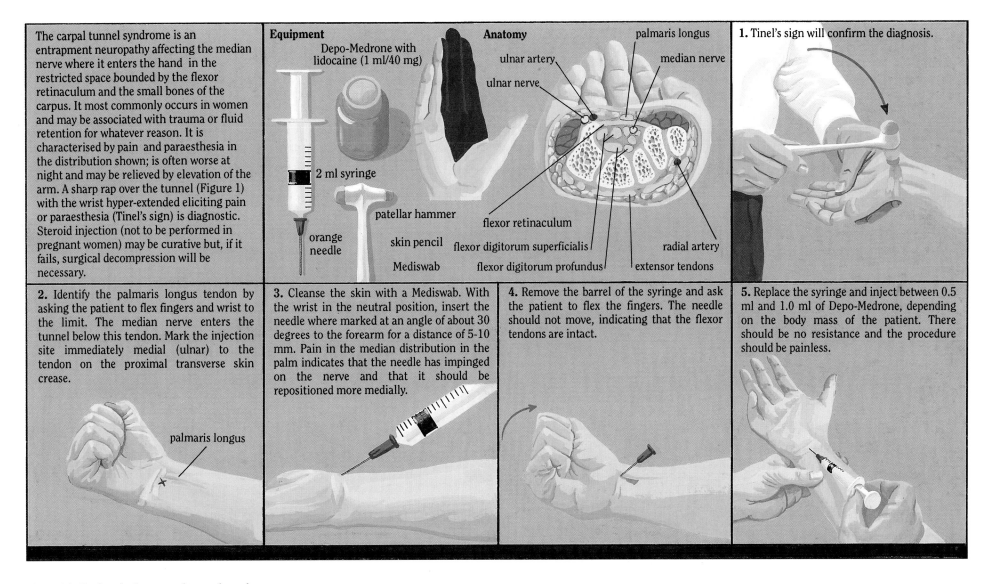

The carpal tunnel syndrome is an entrapment neuropathy affecting the median nerve where it enters the hand in the restricted space bounded by the flexor retinaculum and the small bones of the carpus. It most commonly occurs in women and may be associated with trauma or fluid retention for whatever reason. It is characterised by pain and paraesthesia in the distribution shown; is often worse at night and may be relieved by elevation of the arm. A sharp rap over the tunnel (Figure 1) with the wrist hyper-extended eliciting pain or paraesthesia (Tinel's sign) is diagnostic. Steroid injection (not to be performed in pregnant women) may be curative but, if it fails, surgical decompression will be necessary.

Equipment

Depo-Medrone with lidocaine (1 ml/40 mg)

2 ml syringe

orange needle

patellar hammer

skin pencil

Mediswab

Anatomy

palmaris longus

median nerve

ulnar artery

ulnar nerve

flexor retinaculum

flexor digitorum superficialis

flexor digitorum profundus

radial artery

extensor tendons

1. Tinel's sign will confirm the diagnosis.

2. Identify the palmaris longus tendon by asking the patient to flex fingers and wrist to the limit. The median nerve enters the tunnel below this tendon. Mark the injection site immediately medial (ulnar) to the tendon on the proximal transverse skin crease.

palmaris longus

3. Cleanse the skin with a Mediswab. With the wrist in the neutral position, insert the needle where marked at an angle of about 30 degrees to the forearm for a distance of 5-10 mm. Pain in the median distribution in the palm indicates that the needle has impinged on the nerve and that it should be repositioned more medially.

4. Remove the barrel of the syringe and ask the patient to flex the fingers. The needle should not move, indicating that the flexor tendons are intact.

5. Replace the syringe and inject between 0.5 ml and 1.0 ml of Depo-Medrone, depending on the body mass of the patient. There should be no resistance and the procedure should be painless.

Fig. 7.11. Peri-articular: carpal tunnel syndrome.

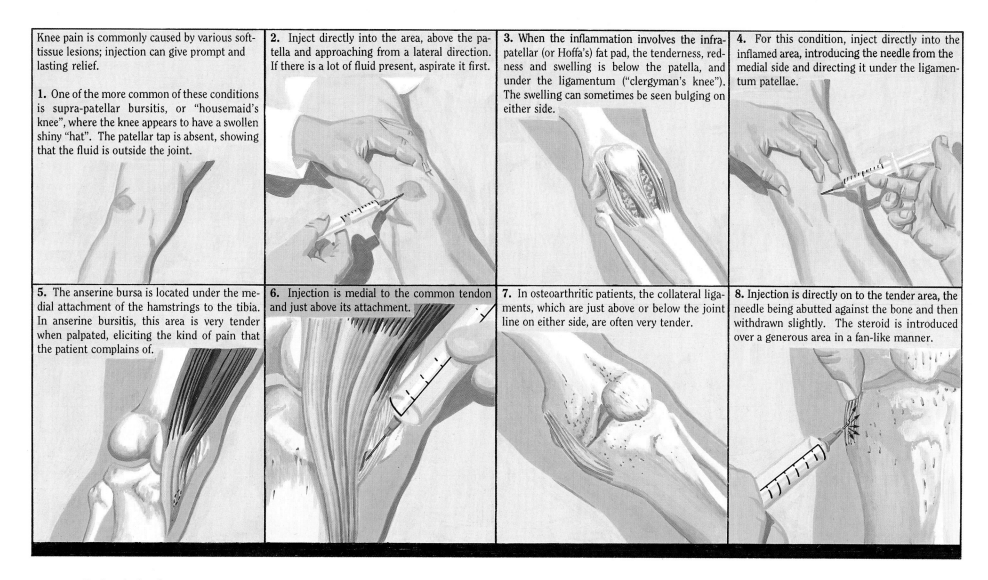

Knee pain is commonly caused by various soft-tissue lesions; injection can give prompt and lasting relief.

1. One of the more common of these conditions is supra-patellar bursitis, or "housemaid's knee", where the knee appears to have a swollen shiny "hat". The patellar tap is absent, showing that the fluid is outside the joint.

2. Inject directly into the area, above the patella and approaching from a lateral direction. If there is a lot of fluid present, aspirate it first.

3. When the inflammation involves the infra-patellar (or Hoffa's) fat pad, the tenderness, redness and swelling is below the patella, and under the ligamentum ("clergyman's knee"). The swelling can sometimes be seen bulging on either side.

4. For this condition, inject directly into the inflamed area, introducing the needle from the medial side and directing it under the ligamentum patellae.

5. The anserine bursa is located under the medial attachment of the hamstrings to the tibia. In anserine bursitis, this area is very tender when palpated, eliciting the kind of pain that the patient complains of.

6. Injection is medial to the common tendon and just above its attachment.

7. In osteoarthritic patients, the collateral ligaments, which are just above or below the joint line on either side, are often very tender.

8. Injection is directly on to the tender area, the needle being abutted against the bone and then withdrawn slightly. The steroid is introduced over a generous area in a fan-like manner.

Fig. 7.12. Peri-articular: knee.

Injections: sclerosant therapy

Sclerotherapy for the primary treatment of venous disorders such as varicose veins and haemorrhoids has been employed for many years as an acceptable alternative to radical surgery. It may readily be undertaken in general practice, thus sparing expensive hospital beds and enabling the patient to remain ambulant (Doran and White 1975). The techniques have changed little over the years.

Sclerotherapy for varicose veins (Fegan's method)
Varicose veins are a common problem in general practice, affecting as many as one in five of the population. They are caused by valvular incompetence in the superficial veins of the lower limb resulting in dilatation and toruosity of the vessels of the saphenous systems. They occur in middle or later life, more commonly in women and may be hereditary in nature but the cause is often not identifiable. They are unsightly and may, in the long term, give rise to thrombophlebitis (especially in men), gravitational eczema, and, eventually, ulceration of the skin of the lower leg.

The rational technique of injection of a sclerosant solution followed by compression was described by Professor W. G. Fegan (Fegan 1963, 1971) and is particularly successful with varicosities which do not extend above the knee. Obliteration is achieved by the injection of an irritant solution into an empty vessel which, when pressure is maintained to occlude the lumen, causes the intimal surfaces of the vein adhere to each other with resulting fibrosis and obstruction. Fraser *et al*. (1985) maintain, however, that prolonged bandaging after injection is not strictly necessary.

Plausible contraindications to sclerotherapy of

varicose veins (although disputed by Fegan (1963)) include previous deep vein thrombosis, obstructive masses in the abdomen or pelvis, pregnancy, and severe varicosities, especially those extending above the knee. The contraceptive pill, if being used, should be stopped for 1 month before treatment.

The traditional sclerosant solutions, now mostly fallen into disuse, were quinine hydrochloride, urethane, and sodium morrhuate. Those commonly used today are shown in Table 7.2. Hydroxypolyethoxydodecane (Polidocanol) has the advantage that it is a local anaesthetic derivative and is thus less painful and, moreover, does not cause tissue necrosis if inadvertently injected outside the vein. The weaker concentration can also be used for the fine needle injection of teleangiectasia (Goldman 1989) although this procedure is not approved for remuneration under current NHS regulations. Furthermore, Polidocanol can only be obtained by prescription on a 'named patient' basis.

Table 7.2. Preparations available for sclerotherapy

Generic name	Proprietary Name	Manufacturer	Availability
Ethanolamine oleate 5 per cent	Ethanolamine Injection	Evans	2 ml, 5 ml ampoule
Sodium tetradecyl	STD	STD Pharmaceutical	0.5 per cent, 2 ml ampoule 1.0 per cent, 2 ml ampoule 3.0 per cent, 2 ml ampoule 5 ml vial
Hydroxypolyethoxydodecane (Polidocanol)	Aetoxysclerol Sclerovein	Laboratoires Pharmaceutique Dexo (Fr.)	0.5 per cent, 2 ml ampoule 2.0 per cent, 2 ml ampoule 3.0 per cent, 2 ml ampoule

References
Doran, F. S. A. and White, M. (1975). A clinical trial designed to discover if the primary treatment of varicose veins should be by Fegan's method or by an operation. *Br. J. Surg.*, **62**, 72–6.

Fegan, W. G. (1963). Continuous compression technique for injecting varicose veins. *Lancet*, **ii**, 109–12.

Fegan, W. G. (1971). The art of bandaging the lower limb. *Br. J. Hosp. Med.*, **5**, 697–8.

Fraser, I. A., Perry, E. P., Hatton, M., and Watkin, D. F. L. (1985) Prolonged bandaging is not required following sclerotherapy of varicose veins. *Br. J. Surg.*, **72**, 488–90.

Goldman, P. M. (1985). Polidocanol (aethoxysklerol) for sclerotherapy of superficial venules and teleangiectasia. *J. Dermatol. Surg. Oncol.*, **15**, 204–9.

Further reading
Fegan, W. G. (1989). Management of vein problems in general practice. *Update*, **1**, 827–30.

Varicose veins are a common problem in general practice, affecting as many as one in ten of the population. They are caused by valvular incompetence in the superficial veins of the lower limb, resulting in dilation and tortuosity of the vessels of the saphenous systems. They occur in middle or later life, are more common in women and may be hereditary. Frequently there is no identifiable cause. They are unsightly and may, in the long term, give rise to thrombophlebitis (especially in men), gravitational eczema and, eventually, ulceration of the skin of the lower leg.

These complications can be averted by the use of sclerotherapy in the early stages and the method of treatment described by Prof. W.G. Fegan (Dublin 1967) is particularly successful with varicosities which do not extend above the knee. It is achieved by the injection of an irritant solution (sodium tetradecyl sulphate 3%) into the empty vessel; the intima of the vein is damaged and, if pressure to occlude the vessel is maintained, the surfaces adhere to each other with resulting fibrosis and obstruction of the lumen.

Contraindications to sclerotherapy

Obstructive mass in the abdomen or pelvis   Pregnancy
Contraceptive pill (should be stopped one month before injection)   Previous deep vein thrombosis
Severe varicosities extending above the knee
Negative Trendelenberg test (see below)

Equipment Sodium tetradecyl sulphate (STD) solution 3%

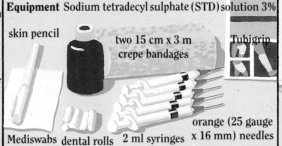

skin pencil

two 15 cm x 3 m crepe bandages

Tubigrip

orange (25 gauge x 16 mm) needles

Mediswabs dental rolls   2 ml syringes

Anatomy   The long saphenous system drains the medial side of the leg and joins the femoral vein through the saphenous opening into the femoral triangle. The short saphenous vein drains the lateral side of the lower leg and enters the popliteal vein in the popliteal fossa.

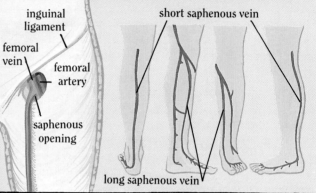

inguinal ligament

short saphenous vein

femoral vein

femoral artery

saphenous opening

long saphenous vein

1. The Trendelenburg test to establish valvular incompetence. Lie the patient down and elevate the affected leg to about 60 degrees.

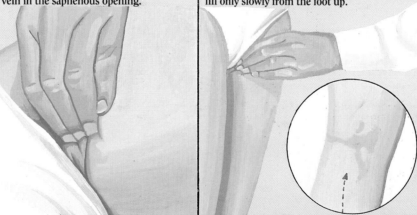

2. When the veins have emptied, apply pressure on the proximal end of the long saphenous vein in the saphenous opening.

3. Maintaining pressure, let the patient stand up again. The veins should remain empty, or fill only slowly from the foot up.

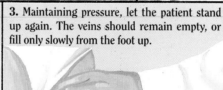

4. Release pressure on the veins; the varicostities should fill rapidly from above down, thus demonstrating incompetence of the valvular system. If they do not do so, look for another cause for varicosities.

Fig. 7.13. Injection of varicose veins—part 1.

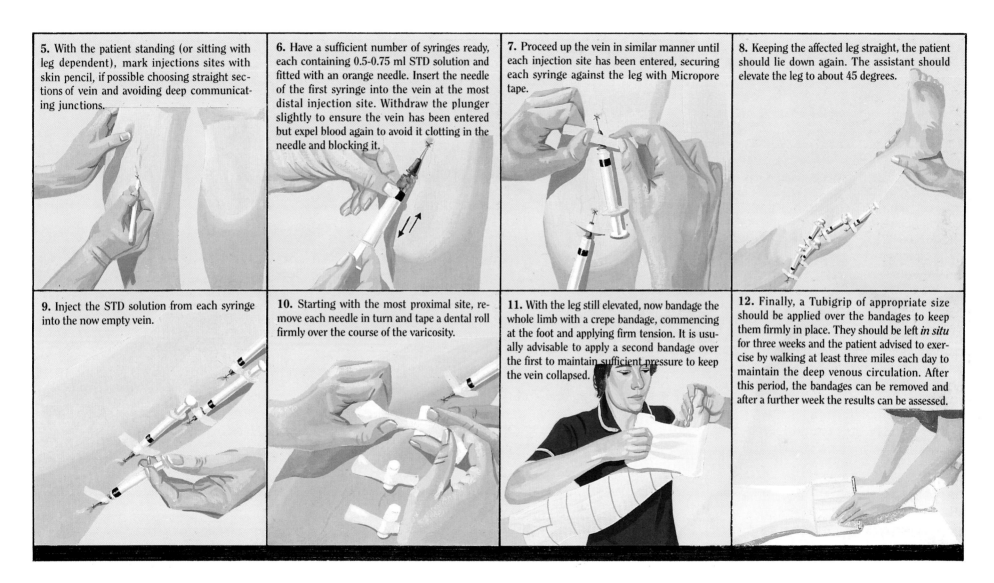

5. With the patient standing (or sitting with leg dependent), mark injections sites with skin pencil, if possible choosing straight sections of vein and avoiding deep communicating junctions.

6. Have a sufficient number of syringes ready, each containing 0.5-0.75 ml STD solution and fitted with an orange needle. Insert the needle of the first syringe into the vein at the most distal injection site. Withdraw the plunger slightly to ensure the vein has been entered but expel blood again to avoid it clotting in the needle and blocking it.

7. Proceed up the vein in similar manner until each injection site has been entered, securing each syringe against the leg with Micropore tape.

8. Keeping the affected leg straight, the patient should lie down again. The assistant should elevate the leg to about 45 degrees.

9. Inject the STD solution from each syringe into the now empty vein.

10. Starting with the most proximal site, remove each needle in turn and tape a dental roll firmly over the course of the varicosity.

11. With the leg still elevated, now bandage the whole limb with a crepe bandage, commencing at the foot and applying firm tension. It is usually advisable to apply a second bandage over the first to maintain sufficient pressure to keep the vein collapsed.

12. Finally, a Tubigrip of appropriate size should be applied over the bandages to keep them firmly in place. They should be left *in situ* for three weeks and the patient advised to exercise by walking at least three miles each day to maintain the deep venous circulation. After this period, the bandages can be removed and after a further week the results can be assessed.

Fig. 7.14. Injection of varicose veins—part 2.

Injection of haemorrhoids

Introduction
Haemorrhoids (piles) are venous dilatations occurring in the superior haemorrhoidal plexus within the anal canal. They may occur in adults of any age and constipation, straining at stool, low-fibre diet, sedentary occupation, etc., are often contributory factors. The usual symptoms are discomfort and bleeding but, in the latter event, it cannot be emphasized too strongly that haemorrhage from higher in the gastrointestinal tract must first be excluded before assuming that the bleeding is resulting merely from piles. Typically, haemorrhoids occur in one or more of the classical sites at 3, 7, and 11 o'clock; first degree piles remain within the anal canal, those of second degree prolapse during defaecation whilst the third degree variety remain chronically prolapsed. The aim of injection is to cause tissue fibrosis at the base of the lesion, thus preventing engorgement and prolapse, rather than thrombosis actually within the vessel. Traditionally, piles are injected with 5 per cent phenol in almond or arachis oil. This substance, which owing to its viscosity and the volume required is, perhaps, not the easiest to use, but has the great advantage that, by virtue of the inherent antiseptic properties of phenol, is most unlikely to give rise to secondary infection.

Further reading
Alexander-Williams, J. (1982). The management of piles. *Br. Med. J..*, **285**, 1137–9.

Goligher, J. (1984) *Surgery of the anus, rectum and colon* (5th edn), pp. 105–13. Balliere Tindall, London.

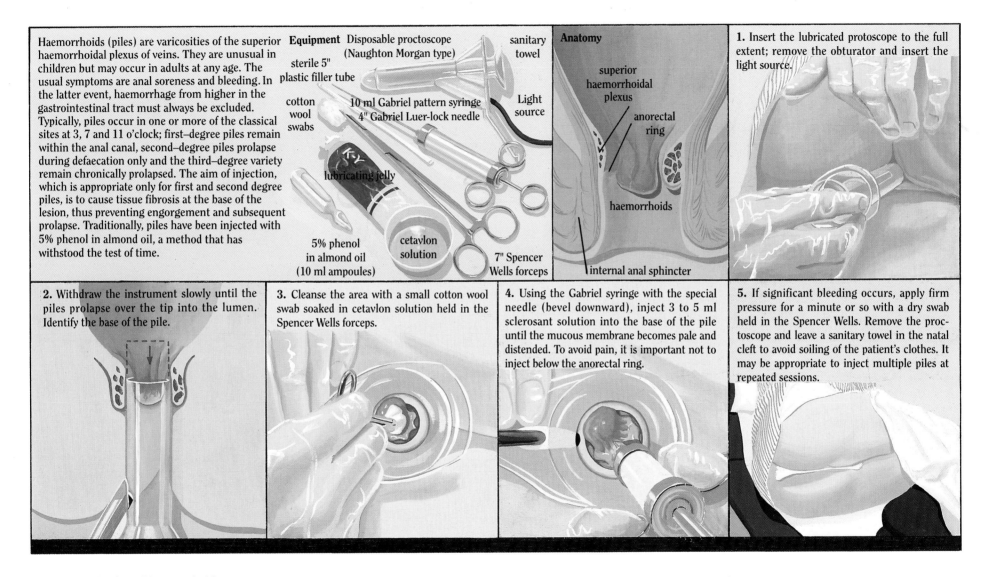

Haemorrhoids (piles) are varicosities of the superior haemorrhoidal plexus of veins. They are unusual in children but may occur in adults at any age. The usual symptoms are anal soreness and bleeding. In the latter event, haemorrhage from higher in the gastrointestinal tract must always be excluded. Typically, piles occur in one or more of the classical sites at 3, 7 and 11 o'clock; first–degree piles remain within the anal canal, second–degree piles prolapse during defaecation only and the third–degree variety remain chronically prolapsed. The aim of injection, which is appropriate only for first and second degree piles, is to cause tissue fibrosis at the base of the lesion, thus preventing engorgement and subsequent prolapse. Traditionally, piles have been injected with 5% phenol in almond oil, a method that has withstood the test of time.

Equipment Disposable proctoscope (Naughton Morgan type)

sterile 5" plastic filler tube

cotton wool swabs

10 ml Gabriel pattern syringe
4" Gabriel Luer-lock needle

sanitary towel

Light source

lubricating jelly

5% phenol in almond oil (10 ml ampoules)

cetavlon solution

7" Spencer Wells forceps

Anatomy

superior haemorrhoidal plexus

anorectal ring

haemorrhoids

internal anal sphincter

1. Insert the lubricated protoscope to the full extent; remove the obturator and insert the light source.

2. Withdraw the instrument slowly until the piles prolapse over the tip into the lumen. Identify the base of the pile.

3. Cleanse the area with a small cotton wool swab soaked in cetavlon solution held in the Spencer Wells forceps.

4. Using the Gabriel syringe with the special needle (bevel downward), inject 3 to 5 ml sclerosant solution into the base of the pile until the mucous membrane becomes pale and distended. To avoid pain, it is important not to inject below the anorectal ring.

5. If significant bleeding occurs, apply firm pressure for a minute or so with a dry swab held in the Spencer Wells. Remove the proctoscope and leave a sanitary towel in the natal cleft to avoid soiling of the patient's clothes. It may be appropriate to inject multiple piles at repeated sessions.

Fig. 7.15. Injection of haemorrhoids.

Aspiration

Introduction

Aspiration of a bursa, cyst, haematoma, or hydrocele is one of the simplest yet most satisfying procedures that can be undertaken in general practice. Again, general principles are important: accurate diagnosis, scrupulous aseptic technique, laboratory examination of the aspirate, prior counselling of the patient, and so on, must all be addressed if errors are to be avoided. Our list is not exhaustive and it should be remembered that some procedures, such as fine needle aspiration biopsy, may not qualify for remuneration under the current regulations. In this section, there may be some reduplication of technique with the procedures listed on pages 55–66 since aspiration may often necessarily precede injection of steroid solutions into joint cavities and bursae.

Further reading

Forrest, A. P. M., Kirkpatrick, J. R., and Roberts, M. M. (1975). Needle aspiration of breast cysts. *Br. Med. J.*, **iii**, 30–1.

Kyle, J., Smith, J. A. R., and Johnston, D. (1992). *Pye's surgical handicraft* (22nd edn.) Butterworth-Heinemann, Oxford.

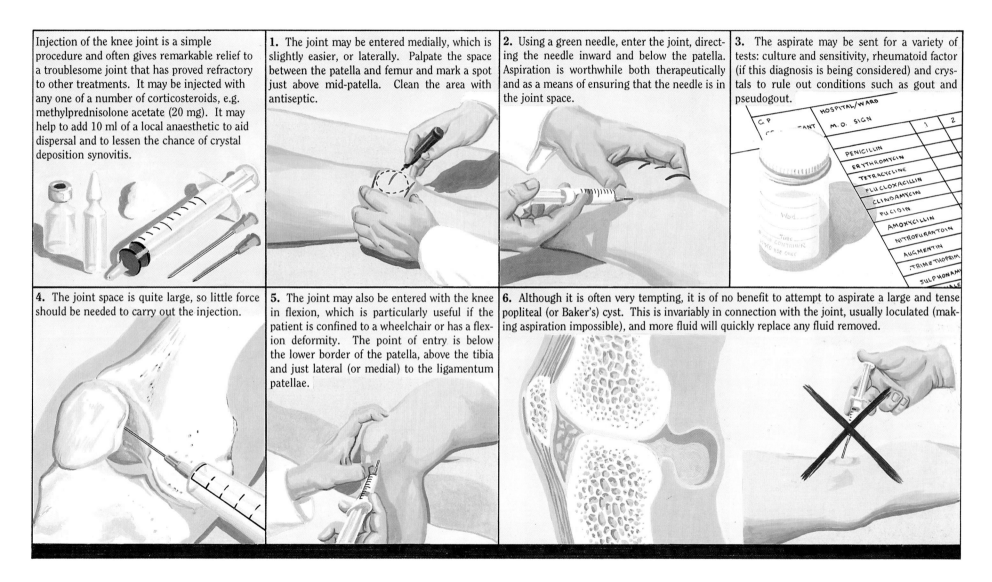

Injection of the knee joint is a simple procedure and often gives remarkable relief to a troublesome joint that has proved refractory to other treatments. It may be injected with any one of a number of corticosteroids, e.g. methylprednisolone acetate (20 mg). It may help to add 10 ml of a local anaesthetic to aid dispersal and to lessen the chance of crystal deposition synovitis.

1. The joint may be entered medially, which is slightly easier, or laterally. Palpate the space between the patella and femur and mark a spot just above mid-patella. Clean the area with antiseptic.

2. Using a green needle, enter the joint, directing the needle inward and below the patella. Aspiration is worthwhile both therapeutically and as a means of ensuring that the needle is in the joint space.

3. The aspirate may be sent for a variety of tests: culture and sensitivity, rheumatoid factor (if this diagnosis is being considered) and crystals to rule out conditions such as gout and pseudogout.

4. The joint space is quite large, so little force should be needed to carry out the injection.

5. The joint may also be entered with the knee in flexion, which is particularly useful if the patient is confined to a wheelchair or has a flexion deformity. The point of entry is below the lower border of the patella, above the tibia and just lateral (or medial) to the ligamentum patellae.

6. Although it is often very tempting, it is of no benefit to attempt to aspirate a large and tense popliteal (or Baker's) cyst. This is invariably in connection with the joint, usually loculated (making aspiration impossible), and more fluid will quickly replace any fluid removed.

Fig. 7.16. Joints: knee.

The elbow is a compound joint comprising the humero-ulnar and the humero-radial articulations. Synovitis may be associated with trauma, infection or osteo-arthritis but perhaps most commonly with rheumatoid arthritis, which will often respond well to the local injection of steroids. In rheumatoid synovitis, quite large effusions may extend anteriorly into the antecubital fossa or laterally from the humero-radial articulation, or both. The connection between the synovial cavity of the joint and the cyst tends to be valvular so, whilst effusions can be aspirated directly, steroid solution injected into the cyst will not enter the joint space. For this reason, it is advisable to use the posterior approach for injection.

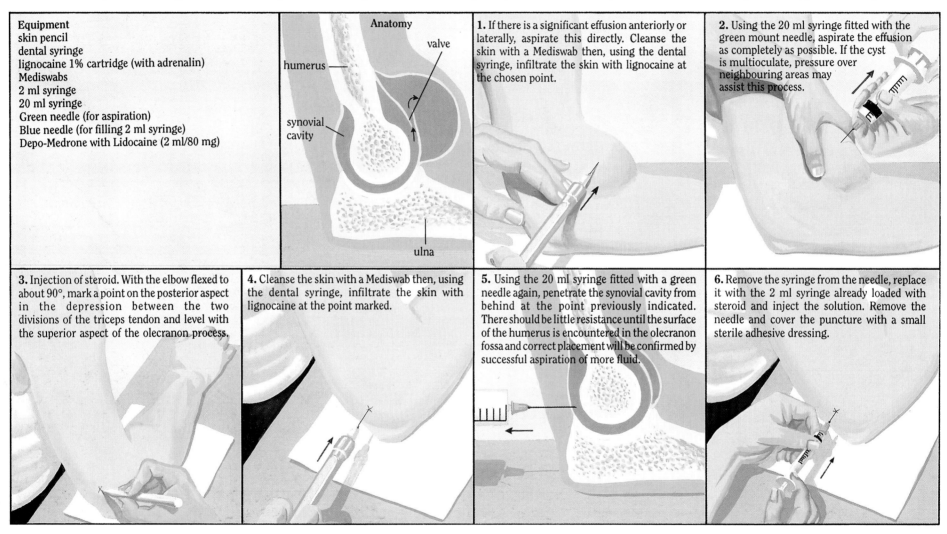

Equipment
skin pencil
dental syringe
lignocaine 1% cartridge (with adrenalin)
Mediswabs
2 ml syringe
20 ml syringe
Green needle (for aspiration)
Blue needle (for filling 2 ml syringe)
Depo-Medrone with Lidocaine (2 ml/80 mg)

Anatomy

valve
humerus
synovial cavity
ulna

1. If there is a significant effusion anteriorly or laterally, aspirate this directly. Cleanse the skin with a Mediswab then, using the dental syringe, infiltrate the skin with lignocaine at the chosen point.

2. Using the 20 ml syringe fitted with the green mount needle, aspirate the effusion as completely as possible. If the cyst is multiloculate, pressure over neighbouring areas may assist this process.

3. Injection of steroid. With the elbow flexed to about 90°, mark a point on the posterior aspect in the depression between the two divisions of the triceps tendon and level with the superior aspect of the olecranon process.

4. Cleanse the skin with a Mediswab then, using the dental syringe, infiltrate the skin with lignocaine at the point marked.

5. Using the 20 ml syringe fitted with a green needle again, penetrate the synovial cavity from behind at the point previously indicated. There should be little resistance until the surface of the humerus is encountered in the olecranon fossa and correct placement will be confirmed by successful aspiration of more fluid.

6. Remove the syringe from the needle, replace it with the 2 ml syringe already loaded with steroid and inject the solution. Remove the needle and cover the puncture with a small sterile adhesive dressing.

Fig. 7.17. Joints: elbow.

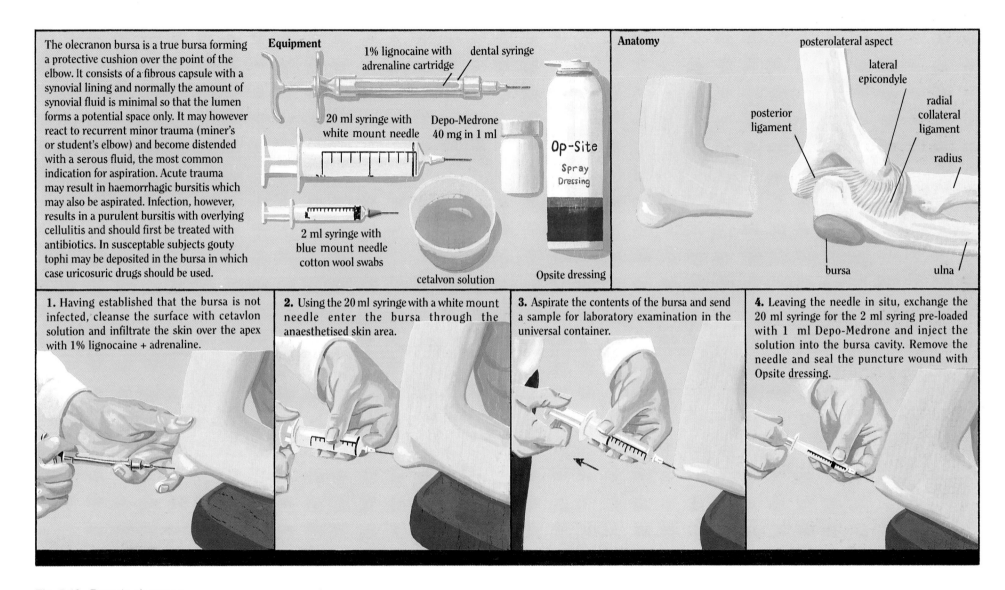

The olecranon bursa is a true bursa forming a protective cushion over the point of the elbow. It consists of a fibrous capsule with a synovial lining and normally the amount of synovial fluid is minimal so that the lumen forms a potential space only. It may however react to recurrent minor trauma (miner's or student's elbow) and become distended with a serous fluid, the most common indication for aspiration. Acute trauma may result in haemorrhagic bursitis which may also be aspirated. Infection, however, results in a purulent bursitis with overlying cellulitis and should first be treated with antibiotics. In susceptable subjects gouty tophi may be deposited in the bursa in which case uricosuric drugs should be used.

Equipment

1% lignocaine with adrenaline cartridge — dental syringe

20 ml syringe with white mount needle

Depo-Medrone 40 mg in 1 ml

Op-Site Spray Dressing

2 ml syringe with blue mount needle cotton wool swabs

cetalvon solution

Opsite dressing

Anatomy

posterolateral aspect

lateral epicondyle

posterior ligament

radial collateral ligament

radius

bursa

ulna

1. Having established that the bursa is not infected, cleanse the surface with cetavlon solution and infiltrate the skin over the apex with 1% lignocaine + adrenaline.

2. Using the 20 ml syringe with a white mount needle enter the bursa through the anaesthetised skin area.

3. Aspirate the contents of the bursa and send a sample for laboratory examination in the universal container.

4. Leaving the needle in situ, exchange the 20 ml syringe for the 2 ml syring pre-loaded with 1 ml Depo-Medrone and inject the solution into the bursa cavity. Remove the needle and seal the puncture wound with Opsite dressing.

Fig. 7.18. Bursae: olecranon.

Inflammation of and effusion into the bursa of the tendo calcaneus (Achilles tendon) is the not uncommon result of athletic over activity and sometimes of ill-fitting footwear. However, it is not infrequently also associated with rheumatoid arthritis, ankylosing spondylitis and Reiter's syndrome and, in the absence of trauma, these conditions should be looked for although their symptoms too will almost certainly benefit from injections of steroids. Furthermore, pain and swelling around the insertion of the Achilles tendon may also be associated with Achilles tendonitis and even with partial avulsion of the tendon from the os calcis, in which instances steroid injection is definitely contraindicated.

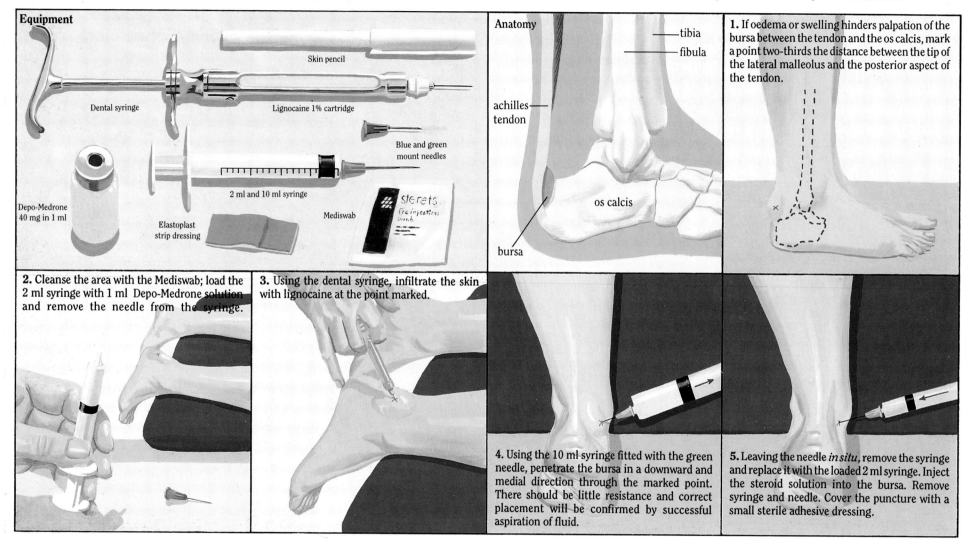

Equipment

Skin pencil

Dental syringe

Lignocaine 1% cartridge

Blue and green mount needles

2 ml and 10 ml syringe

Depo-Medrone 40 mg in 1 ml

Elastoplast strip dressing

Mediswab

Sterets pre-injection swab

Anatomy

tibia

fibula

achilles tendon

os calcis

bursa

1. If oedema or swelling hinders palpation of the bursa between the tendon and the os calcis, mark a point two-thirds the distance between the tip of the lateral malleolus and the posterior aspect of the tendon.

2. Cleanse the area with the Mediswab; load the 2 ml syringe with 1 ml Depo-Medrone solution and remove the needle from the syringe.

3. Using the dental syringe, infiltrate the skin with lignocaine at the point marked.

4. Using the 10 ml syringe fitted with the green needle, penetrate the bursa in a downward and medial direction through the marked point. There should be little resistance and correct placement will be confirmed by successful aspiration of fluid.

5. Leaving the needle *in situ*, remove the syringe and replace it with the loaded 2 ml syringe. Inject the steroid solution into the bursa. Remove syringe and needle. Cover the puncture with a small sterile adhesive dressing.

Fig. 7.19. Bursae: tendo achillis.

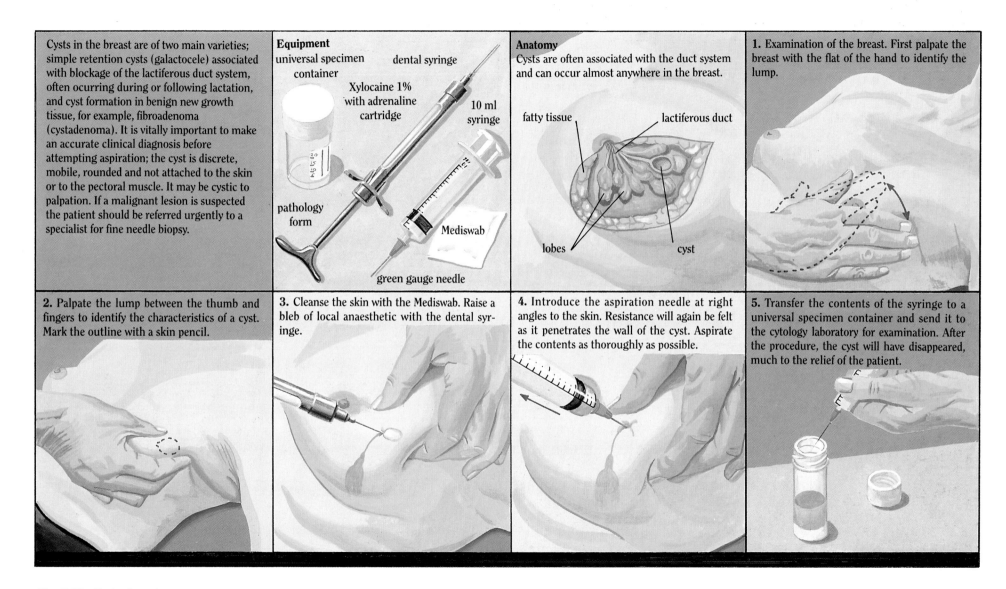

Cysts in the breast are of two main varieties; simple retention cysts (galactocele) associated with blockage of the lactiferous duct system, often ocurring during or following lactation, and cyst formation in benign new growth tissue, for example, fibroadenoma (cystadenoma). It is vitally important to make an accurate clinical diagnosis before attempting aspiration; the cyst is discrete, mobile, rounded and not attached to the skin or to the pectoral muscle. It may be cystic to palpation. If a malignant lesion is suspected the patient should be referred urgently to a specialist for fine needle biopsy.

Equipment
universal specimen container
dental syringe
Xylocaine 1% with adrenaline cartridge
10 ml syringe
pathology form
Mediswab
green gauge needle

Anatomy
Cysts are often associated with the duct system and can occur almost anywhere in the breast.

fatty tissue
lactiferous duct
lobes
cyst

1. Examination of the breast. First palpate the breast with the flat of the hand to identify the lump.

2. Palpate the lump between the thumb and fingers to identify the characteristics of a cyst. Mark the outline with a skin pencil.

3. Cleanse the skin with the Mediswab. Raise a bleb of local anaesthetic with the dental syringe.

4. Introduce the aspiration needle at right angles to the skin. Resistance will again be felt as it penetrates the wall of the cyst. Aspirate the contents as thoroughly as possible.

5. Transfer the contents of the syringe to a universal specimen container and send it to the cytology laboratory for examination. After the procedure, the cyst will have disappeared, much to the relief of the patient.

Fig. 7.20. Cysts: breast.

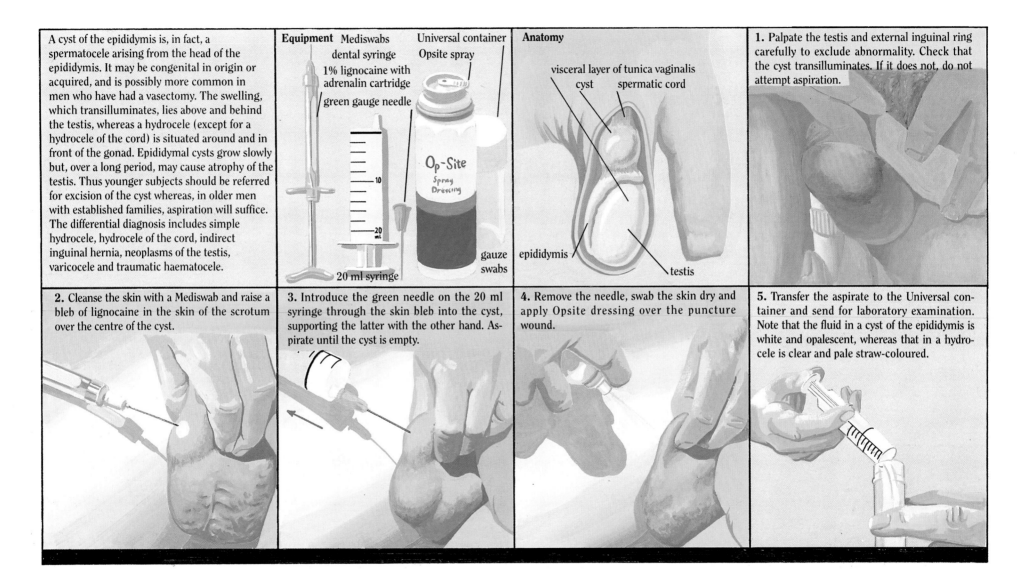

A cyst of the epididymis is, in fact, a spermatocele arising from the head of the epididymis. It may be congenital in origin or acquired, and is possibly more common in men who have had a vasectomy. The swelling, which transilluminates, lies above and behind the testis, whereas a hydrocele (except for a hydrocele of the cord) is situated around and in front of the gonad. Epididymal cysts grow slowly but, over a long period, may cause atrophy of the testis. Thus younger subjects should be referred for excision of the cyst whereas, in older men with established families, aspiration will suffice. The differential diagnosis includes simple hydrocele, hydrocele of the cord, indirect inguinal hernia, neoplasms of the testis, varicocele and traumatic haematocele.

Equipment Mediswabs
dental syringe
1% lignocaine with adrenalin cartridge
green gauge needle
Universal container
Opsite spray

Op-Site Spray Dressing

20 ml syringe
gauze swabs

Anatomy

visceral layer of tunica vaginalis
cyst   spermatic cord
epididymis
testis

1. Palpate the testis and external inguinal ring carefully to exclude abnormality. Check that the cyst transilluminates. If it does not, do not attempt aspiration.

2. Cleanse the skin with a Mediswab and raise a bleb of lignocaine in the skin of the scrotum over the centre of the cyst.

3. Introduce the green needle on the 20 ml syringe through the skin bleb into the cyst, supporting the latter with the other hand. Aspirate until the cyst is empty.

4. Remove the needle, swab the skin dry and apply Opsite dressing over the puncture wound.

5. Transfer the aspirate to the Universal container and send for laboratory examination. Note that the fluid in a cyst of the epididymis is white and opalescent, whereas that in a hydrocele is clear and pale straw-coloured.

Fig. 7.21. Cysts: cyst of epididymis

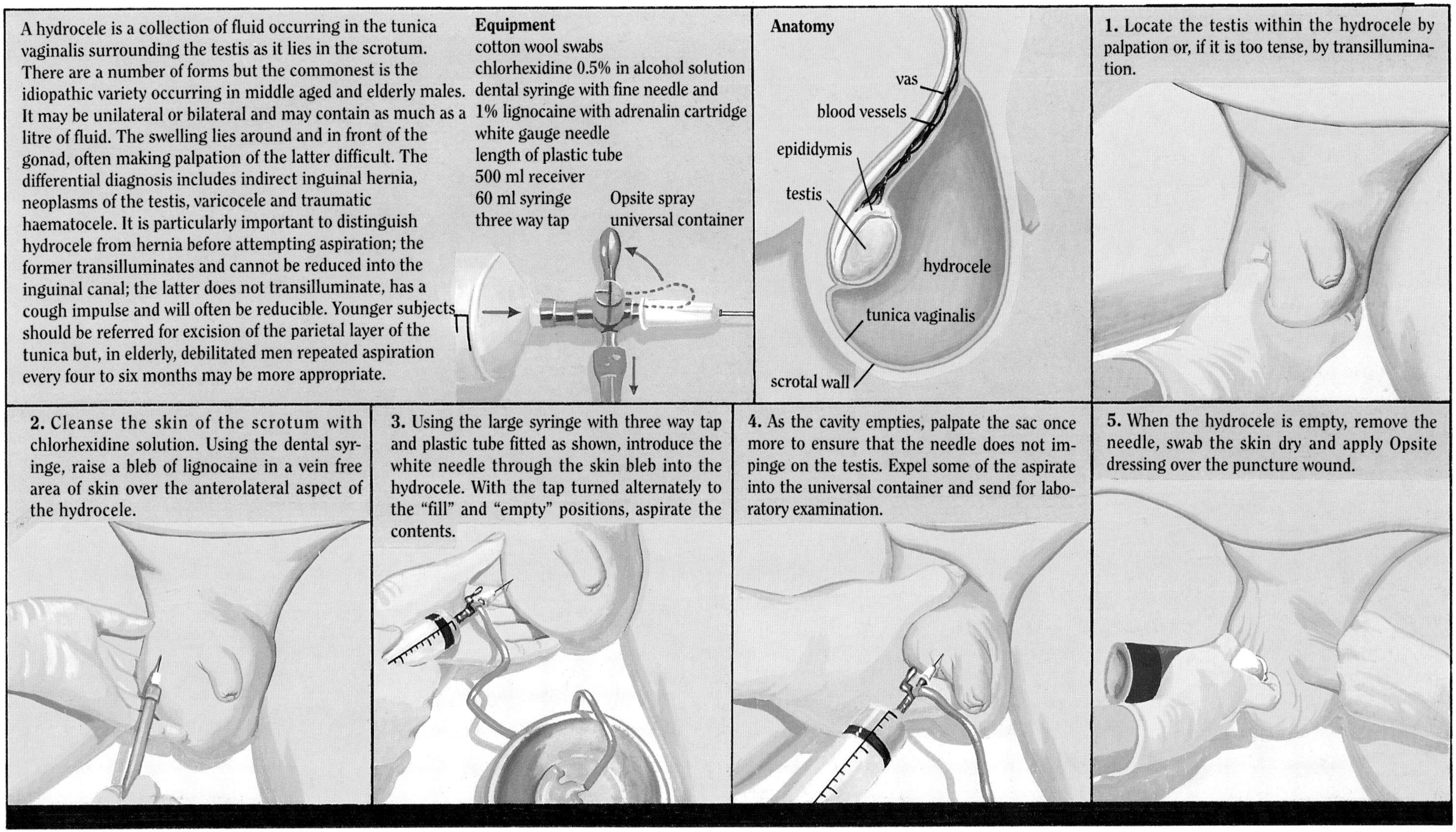

A hydrocele is a collection of fluid occurring in the tunica vaginalis surrounding the testis as it lies in the scrotum. There are a number of forms but the commonest is the idiopathic variety occurring in middle aged and elderly males. It may be unilateral or bilateral and may contain as much as a litre of fluid. The swelling lies around and in front of the gonad, often making palpation of the latter difficult. The differential diagnosis includes indirect inguinal hernia, neoplasms of the testis, varicocele and traumatic haematocele. It is particularly important to distinguish hydrocele from hernia before attempting aspiration; the former transilluminates and cannot be reduced into the inguinal canal; the latter does not transilluminate, has a cough impulse and will often be reducible. Younger subjects should be referred for excision of the parietal layer of the tunica but, in elderly, debilitated men repeated aspiration every four to six months may be more appropriate.

Equipment
cotton wool swabs
chlorhexidine 0.5% in alcohol solution
dental syringe with fine needle and
1% lignocaine with adrenalin cartridge
white gauge needle
length of plastic tube
500 ml receiver
60 ml syringe   Opsite spray
three way tap   universal container

Anatomy

vas
blood vessels
epididymis
testis
hydrocele
tunica vaginalis
scrotal wall

1. Locate the testis within the hydrocele by palpation or, if it is too tense, by transillumination.

2. Cleanse the skin of the scrotum with chlorhexidine solution. Using the dental syringe, raise a bleb of lignocaine in a vein free area of skin over the anterolateral aspect of the hydrocele.

3. Using the large syringe with three way tap and plastic tube fitted as shown, introduce the white needle through the skin bleb into the hydrocele. With the tap turned alternately to the "fill" and "empty" positions, aspirate the contents.

4. As the cavity empties, palpate the sac once more to ensure that the needle does not impinge on the testis. Expel some of the aspirate into the universal container and send for laboratory examination.

5. When the hydrocele is empty, remove the needle, swab the skin dry and apply Opsite dressing over the puncture wound.

Fig. 7.22. Other: hydrocele.

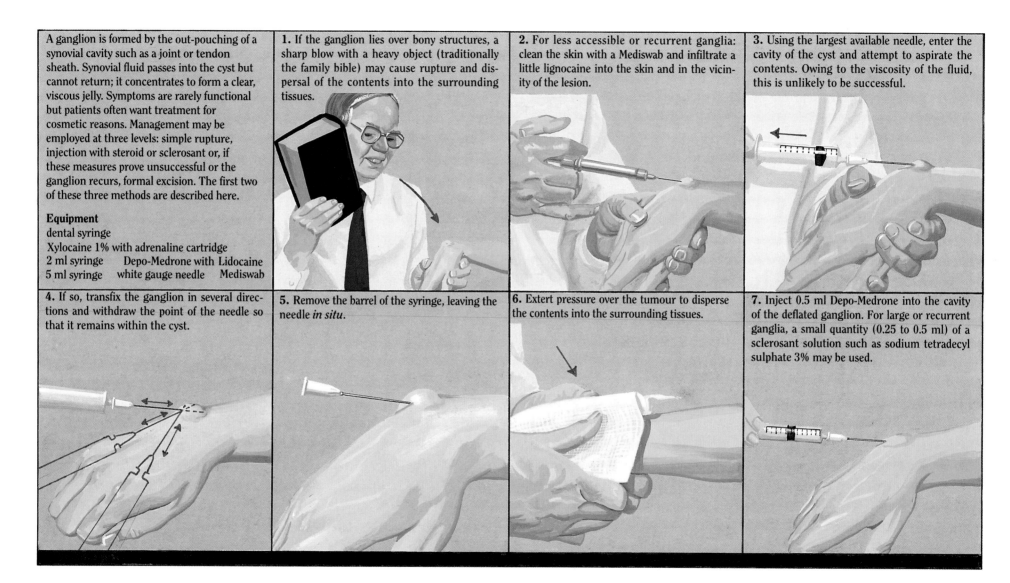

A ganglion is formed by the out-pouching of a synovial cavity such as a joint or tendon sheath. Synovial fluid passes into the cyst but cannot return; it concentrates to form a clear, viscous jelly. Symptoms are rarely functional but patients often want treatment for cosmetic reasons. Management may be employed at three levels: simple rupture, injection with steroid or sclerosant or, if these measures prove unsuccessful or the ganglion recurs, formal excision. The first two of these three methods are described here.

Equipment
dental syringe
Xylocaine 1% with adrenaline cartridge
2 ml syringe   Depo-Medrone with Lidocaine
5 ml syringe   white gauge needle   Mediswab

1. If the ganglion lies over bony structures, a sharp blow with a heavy object (traditionally the family bible) may cause rupture and dispersal of the contents into the surrounding tissues.

2. For less accessible or recurrent ganglia: clean the skin with a Mediswab and infiltrate a little lignocaine into the skin and in the vicinity of the lesion.

3. Using the largest available needle, enter the cavity of the cyst and attempt to aspirate the contents. Owing to the viscosity of the fluid, this is unlikely to be successful.

4. If so, transfix the ganglion in several directions and withdraw the point of the needle so that it remains within the cyst.

5. Remove the barrel of the syringe, leaving the needle *in situ*.

6. Extert pressure over the tumour to disperse the contents into the surrounding tissues.

7. Inject 0.5 ml Depo-Medrone into the cavity of the deflated ganglion. For large or recurrent ganglia, a small quantity (0.25 to 0.5 ml) of a sclerosant solution such as sodium tetradecyl sulphate 3% may be used.

Fig. 7.23. Other: ganglion.

Incision

Introduction

'If there be pus, let it out!' – so runs the time honoured adage, no less true in these days of ever more potent and versatile antibiotics. Once pus has formed, the best that chemotherapy can do is to render the abscess sterile or prevent surrounding cellulitis and the more distant spread of infection. Although abscesses of all descriptions appear to qualify under the minor surgery regulations for treatment in general practice, the author has grave reservations concerning the advisability of tackling those of a major nature (for example, abscesses in the breast, axilla, and perineum or big carbuncles) unless safe and effective general anaesthesia is available. Since this is not usually the case in most practices, these particular procedures have not been addressed. In the case of less extensive superficial infections, however, the overlying dermis may already be necrotic and, thus, insensitive to the knife. In this instance, a patient may prefer immediate incision and drainage to a time-consuming hospital attendance. Local infiltration of anaesthetic solutions should not be practised when treating infected lesions, firstly, owing to the risk of provoking local cellulitis and, secondly, because the analgesic effect is, in any case, greatly diminished in the presence of inflammation. Peripheral infections of the hands and feet, however, should present no problem since adequate and safe analgesia can be achieved by the use of the appropriate regional blocks (see Chapter 3).

Further reading

Kyle, J., Smith, J. A. R., and Johnston, D. (1992). *Pye's surgical handicraft* (22nd edn). Butterworth-Heinemann, Oxford.

Snook, R. (1971). Minor surgery: the hand. *Update Plus*, **1**, 449–54, 543–53.

Snook, R. (1972). Minor surgery: septic lesions. *Update*, **4**, 89–92.

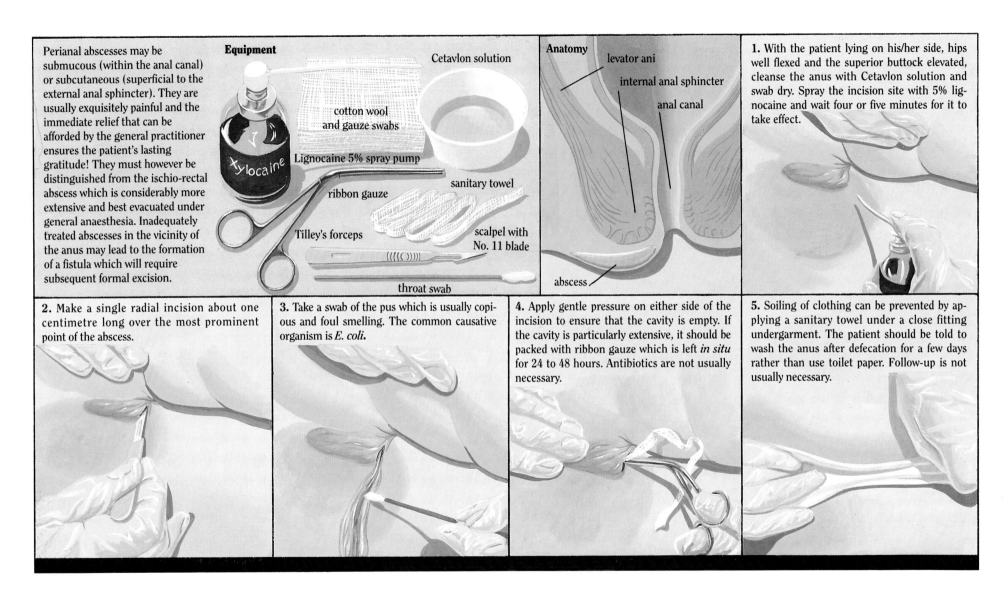

Perianal abscesses may be submucous (within the anal canal) or subcutaneous (superficial to the external anal sphincter). They are usually exquisitely painful and the immediate relief that can be afforded by the general practitioner ensures the patient's lasting gratitude! They must however be distinguished from the ischio-rectal abscess which is considerably more extensive and best evacuated under general anaesthesia. Inadequately treated abscesses in the vicinity of the anus may lead to the formation of a fistula which will require subsequent formal excision.

Equipment

cotton wool and gauze swabs

Cetavlon solution

Lignocaine 5% spray pump

ribbon gauze

sanitary towel

Tilley's forceps

scalpel with No. 11 blade

throat swab

Anatomy

levator ani

internal anal sphincter

anal canal

abscess

1. With the patient lying on his/her side, hips well flexed and the superior buttock elevated, cleanse the anus with Cetavlon solution and swab dry. Spray the incision site with 5% lignocaine and wait four or five minutes for it to take effect.

2. Make a single radial incision about one centimetre long over the most prominent point of the abscess.

3. Take a swab of the pus which is usually copious and foul smelling. The common causative organism is *E. coli.*

4. Apply gentle pressure on either side of the incision to ensure that the cavity is empty. If the cavity is particularly extensive, it should be packed with ribbon gauze which is left *in situ* for 24 to 48 hours. Antibiotics are not usually necessary.

5. Soiling of clothing can be prevented by applying a sanitary towel under a close fitting undergarment. The patient should be told to wash the anus after defecation for a few days rather than use toilet paper. Follow-up is not usually necessary.

Fig. 7.24. Abscesses: peri-anal.

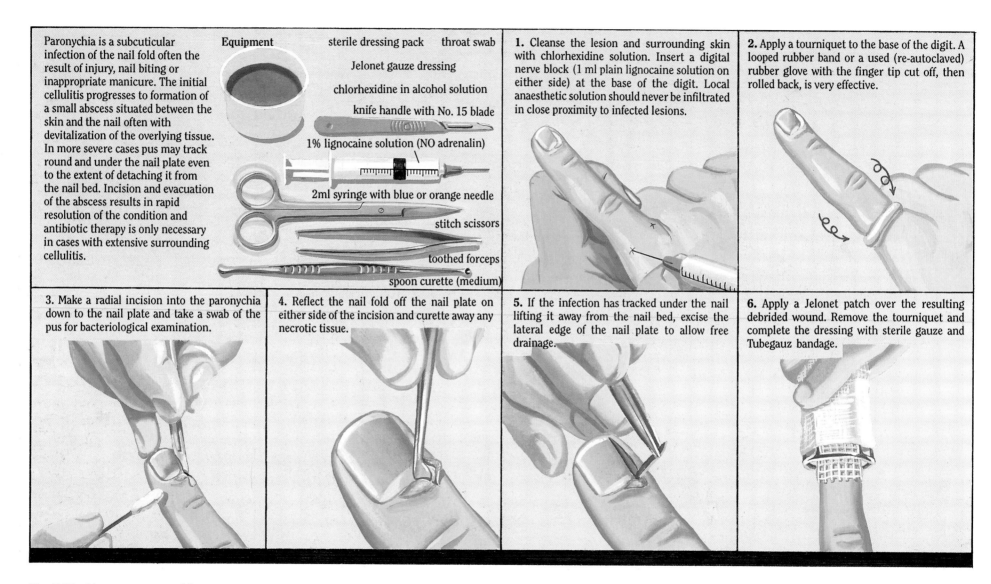

Paronychia is a subcuticular infection of the nail fold often the result of injury, nail biting or inappropriate manicure. The initial cellulitis progresses to formation of a small abscess situated between the skin and the nail often with devitalization of the overlying tissue. In more severe cases pus may track round and under the nail plate even to the extent of detaching it from the nail bed. Incision and evacuation of the abscess results in rapid resolution of the condition and antibiotic therapy is only necessary in cases with extensive surrounding cellulitis.

Equipment   sterile dressing pack   throat swab

Jelonet gauze dressing

chlorhexidine in alcohol solution

knife handle with No. 15 blade

1% lignocaine solution (NO adrenalin)

2ml syringe with blue or orange needle

stitch scissors

toothed forceps

spoon curette (medium)

1. Cleanse the lesion and surrounding skin with chlorhexidine solution. Insert a digital nerve block (1 ml plain lignocaine solution on either side) at the base of the digit. Local anaesthetic solution should never be infiltrated in close proximity to infected lesions.

2. Apply a tourniquet to the base of the digit. A looped rubber band or a used (re-autoclaved) rubber glove with the finger tip cut off, then rolled back, is very effective.

3. Make a radial incision into the paronychia down to the nail plate and take a swab of the pus for bacteriological examination.

4. Reflect the nail fold off the nail plate on either side of the incision and curette away any necrotic tissue.

5. If the infection has tracked under the nail lifting it away from the nail bed, excise the lateral edge of the nail plate to allow free drainage.

6. Apply a Jelonet patch over the resulting debrided wound. Remove the tourniquet and complete the dressing with sterile gauze and Tubegauz bandage.

Fig. 7.25. Abscesses: paronychia.

Terminal pulp abscesses are frequently the result of accidental puncture of the tip of a digit with a thorn or splinter but a foreign body is not retained. The infection is characterised by throbbing pain with swelling and inflammation around the site of puncture. Pain is particularly severe owing to division of the pulp into restricted fascial compartments and extensive innervation of the finger tips. Collar stud abscesses are prone to develop in this situation and it is important to ensure that drainage is complete and necrotic tissue excised as far as possible. Effective incision and debridement of the abscess results in rapid resolution but complementary antibiotic therapy is advisable to prevent osteomyelitis of the terminal phalanx.

Equipment
sterile dressing pack
chlorhexidine in alcohol solution
2 ml syringe with blue and orange needles
2% lignocaine solution (NO adrenaline)
tourniquet
knife handle with no. 15 blade
throat swab
fine silver probe
spoon curette (medium/small)
fine-toothed forceps
stitch scissors
sterile ribbon gauze (25 mm)
Tubegauz bandage

1. Cleanse the lesion and surrounding skin with chlorhexidine solution. Insert a digital nerve block as described in Fig. 7.33, and apply a tourniquet. Local anaesthetic solution should *never* be infiltrated in close proximity to the infected lesion.

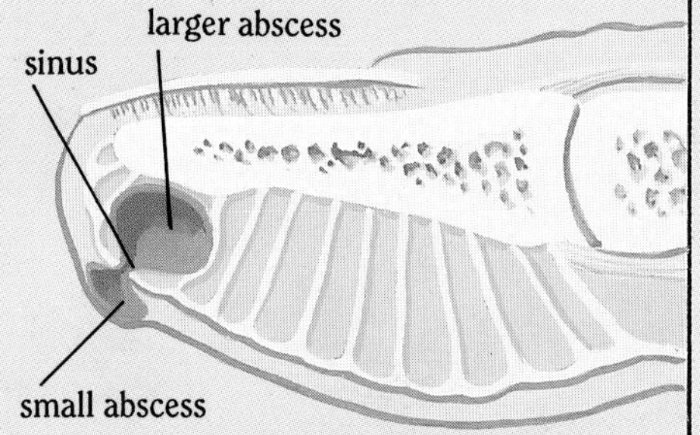

larger abscess
sinus
small abscess

2. Make an inverted J-shaped incision on the side of the terminal pulp, where the abscess is pointing.

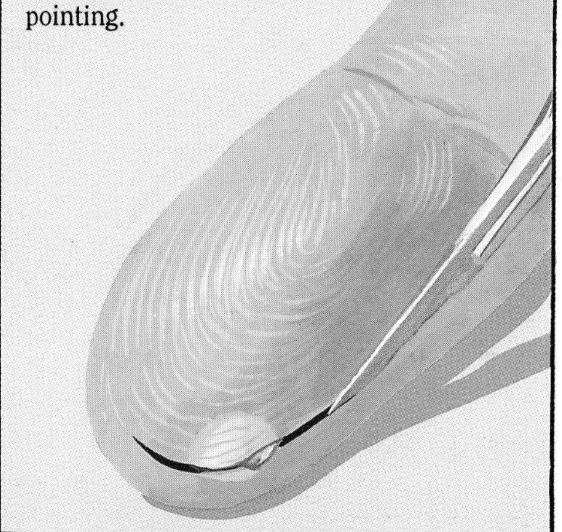

3. Take a swab of any frank pus for bacteriological examination.

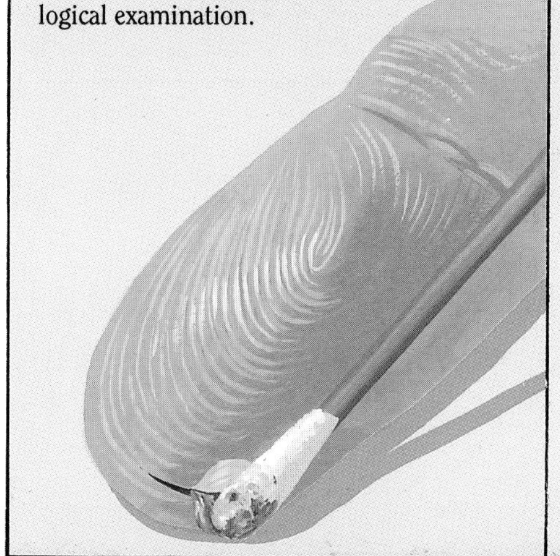

4. Explore the wound with the probe to identify a collar stud sinus.

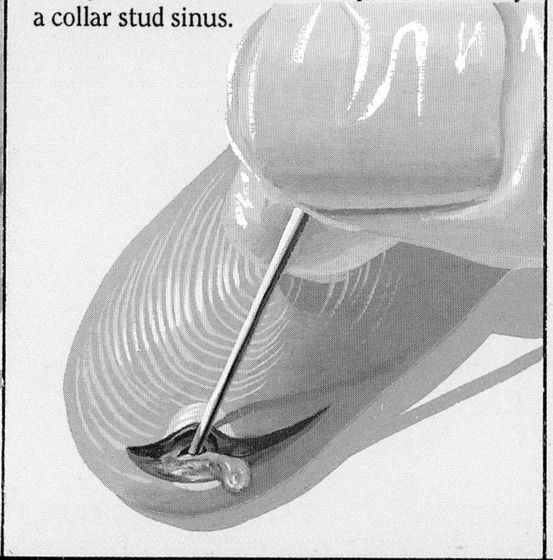

5. If a sinus is found, extend the original incision more deeply to lay open the deep cavity.

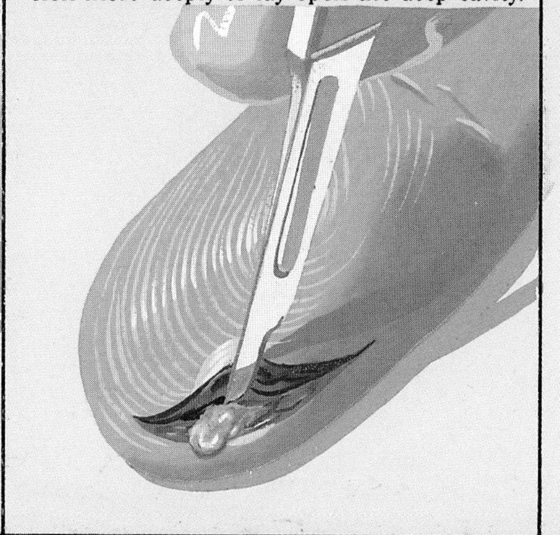

6. Curette or excise necrotic tissue from the cavity and track as throughly as possible. Reapproximate the skin edges. Bandage the finger tip with sterile ribbon gauze and complete the dressing with Tubegauz bandage. Remove the tourniquet and advise the patient to use an arm sling until redressing in two or three days.

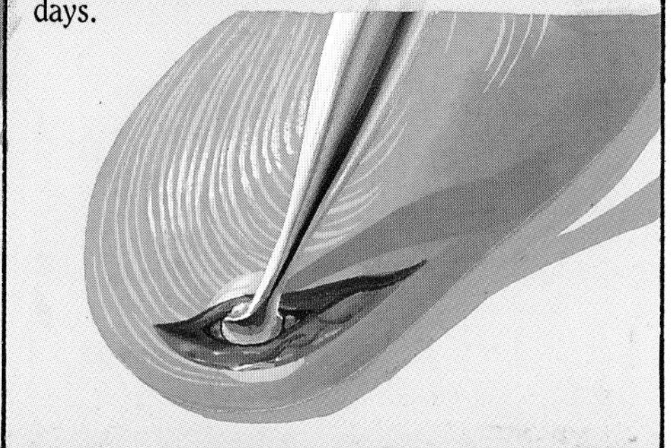

Fig. 7.26. Abscesses: terminal pulp (collar stud) abscess.

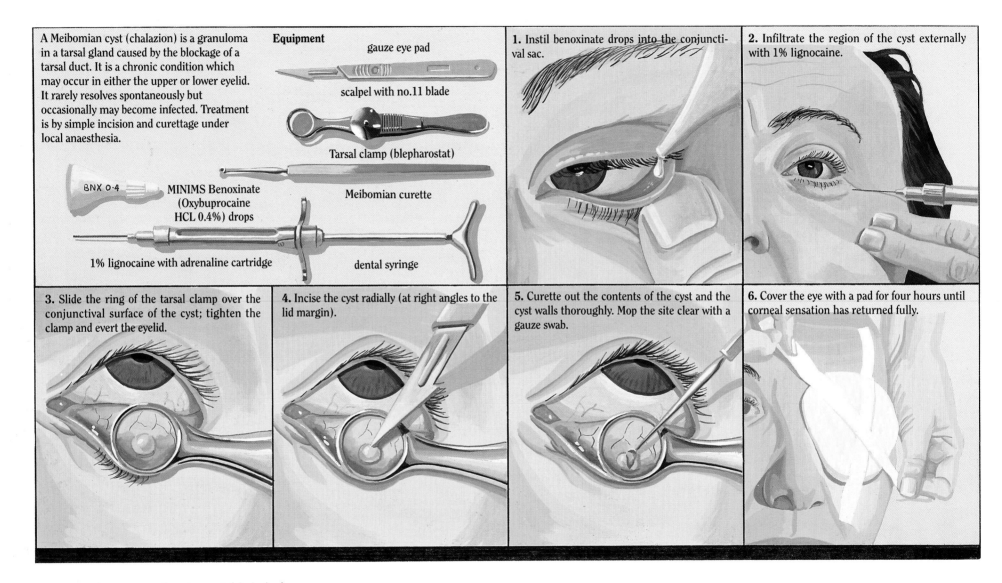

A Meibomian cyst (chalazion) is a granuloma in a tarsal gland caused by the blockage of a tarsal duct. It is a chronic condition which may occur in either the upper or lower eyelid. It rarely resolves spontaneously but occasionally may become infected. Treatment is by simple incision and curettage under local anaesthesia.

Equipment
gauze eye pad
scalpel with no.11 blade
Tarsal clamp (blepharostat)
Meibomian curette
dental syringe

BNX 0·4 — MINIMS Benoxinate (Oxybuprocaine HCL 0.4%) drops

1% lignocaine with adrenaline cartridge

1. Instil benoxinate drops into the conjunctival sac.

2. Infiltrate the region of the cyst externally with 1% lignocaine.

3. Slide the ring of the tarsal clamp over the conjunctival surface of the cyst; tighten the clamp and evert the eyelid.

4. Incise the cyst radially (at right angles to the lid margin).

5. Curette out the contents of the cyst and the cyst walls thoroughly. Mop the site clear with a gauze swab.

6. Cover the eye with a pad for four hours until corneal sensation has returned fully.

Fig. 7.27. Abscesses: meibomian cyst (chalazion).

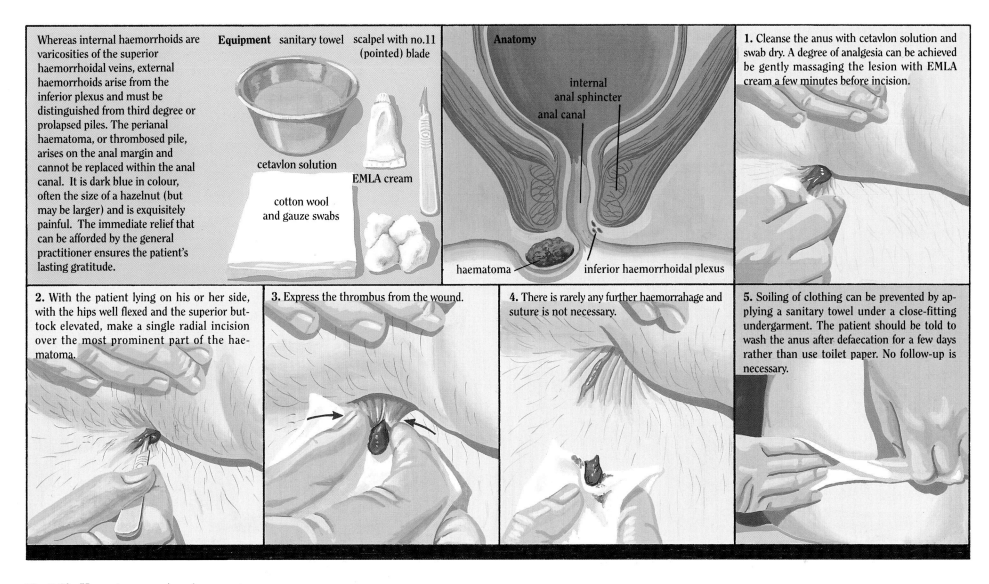

Whereas internal haemorrhoids are varicosities of the superior haemorrhoidal veins, external haemorrhoids arise from the inferior plexus and must be distinguished from third degree or prolapsed piles. The perianal haematoma, or thrombosed pile, arises on the anal margin and cannot be replaced within the anal canal. It is dark blue in colour, often the size of a hazelnut (but may be larger) and is exquisitely painful. The immediate relief that can be afforded by the general practitioner ensures the patient's lasting gratitude.

Equipment sanitary towel scalpel with no.11 (pointed) blade

cetavlon solution

EMLA cream

cotton wool and gauze swabs

Anatomy

internal anal sphincter

anal canal

haematoma

inferior haemorrhoidal plexus

1. Cleanse the anus with cetavlon solution and swab dry. A degree of analgesia can be achieved be gently massaging the lesion with EMLA cream a few minutes before incision.

2. With the patient lying on his or her side, with the hips well flexed and the superior buttock elevated, make a single radial incision over the most prominent part of the haematoma.

3. Express the thrombus from the wound.

4. There is rarely any further haemorrhage and suture is not necessary.

5. Soiling of clothing can be prevented by applying a sanitary towel under a close-fitting undergarment. The patient should be told to wash the anus after defaecation for a few days rather than use toilet paper. No follow-up is necessary.

Fig. 7.28. Haematoma: peri-anal.

Excisions

Introduction

The excision of dermatological lesions either for therapeutic, diagnostic, or cosmetic reasons, will be the nearest approach to formal surgery that the general practitioner will undertake in his day to day work. The principles involved have been discussed in some detail with regard to infection control, analgesia, and technique in Chapters 2, 3, and 5, respectively and a variety of more specific procedures are described in this section. More recently, (McWilliam *et al*. 1991; Williams *et al*. 1991) concern has been expressed concerning both the accuracy of diagnosis of dermatological lesions by general practitioners and submission of specimens by them for histological examination. There are, of course, medico-legal implications in this (Chapter 4) so a rule of thumb should be to submit all excised specimens, with full details regarding location, provisional diagnosis, and so on, for histological examination. It is equally important (except in the case of diagnostic biopsies) to ensure that lesions are completely excised and, wherever possible, a small margin of normal surrounding tissue should be included. Shave, punch, and excision biopsy methods are also described.

Ingrowing toenails are another common problem and one sometimes referred on to general practitioners by chiropodists. Variations in technique are legion (see Further reading) and the three main approaches, wedge resection with either complete excision or chemical ablation of the germinal matrix are described together with complete ablation (Zadik 1950) a technique more appropriate for recurrent infections.

References

McWilliam, L. J., Knox, F., Wilkinson, N., and Oogarah, P. (1991). Performance of skin biopsies by general practitioners. *Br. Med. J.*, **303**, 1177–8.

Williams, R. B., Burdge, A. H., and Lewis Jones, S. (1991). Skin biopsy in general practice. *Br. Med. J.*., **303**, 1179–80.

Zadik, F. R. (1950). Obliteration of the nail bed of the great toe without shortening the terminal phalanx. *J. Bone. Joint Surg.*, **32B**, 66–7.

Further reading

Cracknell, I. and Mead, M. (1991). Excisions: lipomata. *Update*, 42, 869–74.

Cracknell, I. and Mead, M. (1991). Excisions: papillomata, skin tags, moles and verrucae. *Update*, **42**, 1085–90.

Snook, R. (1971). Minor surgery: sebaceous cysts and other lesions. *Update Plus*, **1**, 655–61.

Ingrowing toenails

Cameron, P. F. (1981). Ingrowing toe nails—an evaluation of two treatments. *Br. Med. J.*, **283**, 821–2.

Cracknell, I. (1992). Phenolisation of the ingrowing toenail. *Update*, **44**, 1174–6.

Cracknell, I. and Mead, M. (1991). Excision of the ingrowing toenail. *Update*, **42**, 465–71.

Fowler, A. W. (1976). Ingrowing toe nails. *Br. Med. J.*, **ii**, 815–16.

Palmer, B. V. and Stevenson, D. L. (1976). Modified operation for ingrowing toe nails. *Br. Med. J.*, **ii**, 367 (letter).

Sykes, P. A. (1986). Ingrowing toe nails: time for critical appraisal? *J. Roy. Coll. Surg. Edinb.*, **31**, 300–4.

Wallace, W. A., Milne, D. D., and Andrew, T. T. (1979) Gutter treatment for ingrowing toenails. *Br. Med. J.*, **ii**, 168–71.

Winograd, A. M. (1929). A modification in the technique of operation for ingrowing toe nail. *J. Am. Med. Ass.*, **92**, 229–30.

Skin biopsy

Healsmith, M. and Graham-Brown, R. (1991). Punch biopsy of skin lesions. *Update*, **43**, 797–800.

Sebaceous cysts result from the blockage of the duct of a sebaceous gland and subsequent continued secretion of sebum. They are often multiple and commonly occur on the scalp, face, back, neck and scrotum. They are connected to the skin by the duct (the punctum can often be seen) but rarely to any underlying structure, so excision under local analgesia is usually a simple operation. The removal of a cyst on a patient's scalp is illustrated here.

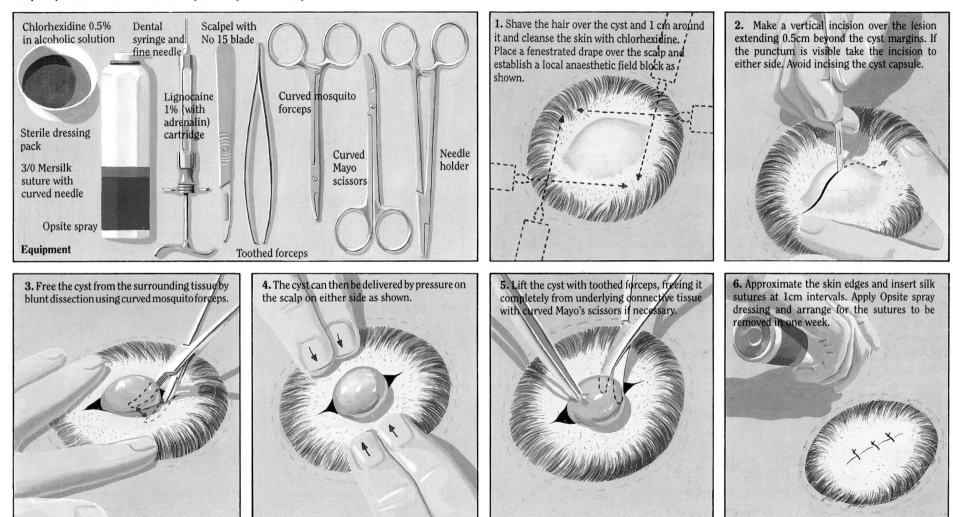

Chlorhexidine 0.5% in alcoholic solution

Dental syringe and fine needle

Scalpel with No 15 blade

Lignocaine 1% (with adrenalin) cartridge

Sterile dressing pack

3/0 Mersilk suture with curved needle

Opsite spray

Curved mosquito forceps

Curved Mayo scissors

Needle holder

Toothed forceps

Equipment

1. Shave the hair over the cyst and 1 cm around it and cleanse the skin with chlorhexidine. Place a fenestrated drape over the scalp and establish a local anaesthetic field block as shown.

2. Make a vertical incision over the lesion extending 0.5cm beyond the cyst margins. If the punctum is visible take the incision to either side. Avoid incising the cyst capsule.

3. Free the cyst from the surrounding tissue by blunt dissection using curved mosquito forceps.

4. The cyst can then be delivered by pressure on the scalp on either side as shown.

5. Lift the cyst with toothed forceps, freeing it completely from underlying connective tissue with curved Mayo's scissors if necessary.

6. Approximate the skin edges and insert silk sutures at 1cm intervals. Apply Opsite spray dressing and arrange for the sutures to be removed in one week.

Fig. 7.29. Tumours: sebaceous cyst.

Lipomata are slowly-growing benign fatty tumours that may be encapsulated or diffuse. They are often multiple and can occur on almost any part of the body. They are very variable in size, soft, mobile, often irregular in outline and sometimes give a false impression of fluctuation. When subcutaneous they can usually be removed under local anaesthetic without difficulty but some patients may prefer to keep an inoffensive swelling rather than accept the inevitable linear scar that results from excision.

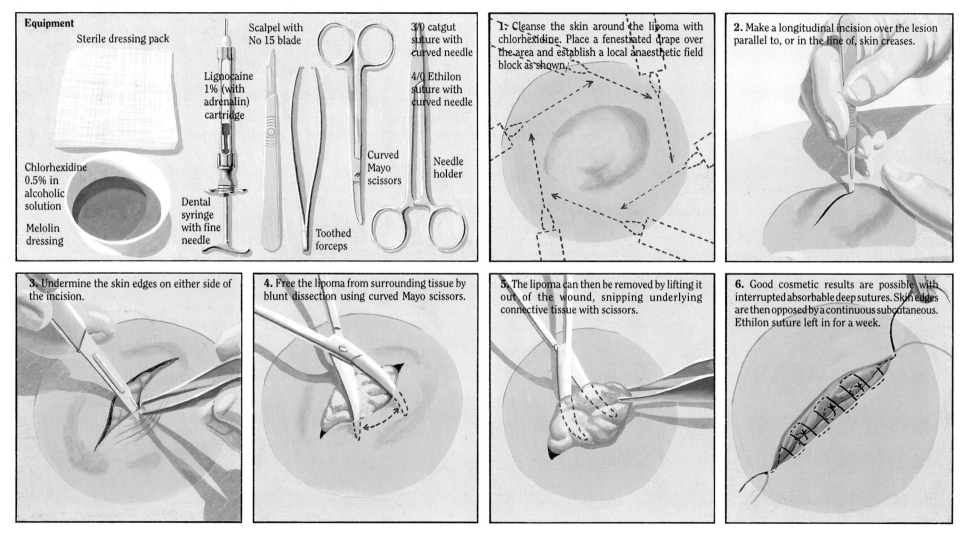

Equipment
Sterile dressing pack

Chlorhexidine 0.5% in alcoholic solution

Melolin dressing

Lignocaine 1% (with adrenalin) cartridge

Dental syringe with fine needle

Scalpel with No 15 blade

Toothed forceps

Curved Mayo scissors

3/0 catgut suture with curved needle

4/0 Ethilon suture with curved needle

Needle holder

1. Cleanse the skin around the lipoma with chlorhexidine. Place a fenestrated drape over the area and establish a local anaesthetic field block as shown.

2. Make a longitudinal incision over the lesion parallel to, or in the line of, skin creases.

3. Undermine the skin edges on either side of the incision.

4. Free the lipoma from surrounding tissue by blunt dissection using curved Mayo scissors.

5. The lipoma can then be removed by lifting it out of the wound, snipping underlying connective tissue with scissors.

6. Good cosmetic results are possible with interrupted absorbable deep sutures. Skin edges are then opposed by a continuous subcutaneous Ethilon suture left in for a week.

Fig. 7.30. Tumours: lipoma.

Dermatofibromata are small, reddish-brown raised nodules, often occuring on exposed surfaces on the body. They are invariably benign but removal is often requested for cosmetic reasons and the method described here may be used as a model for excision procedures in general. To obtain acceptable cosmetic results, incisions should be made in the line of natural skin creases and the wound should be repaired using fine non-absorbable suture material. Always send excised specimens for histological examination, having taken care to preserve a narrow surround of normal skin on either side to confirm that removal has been complete.

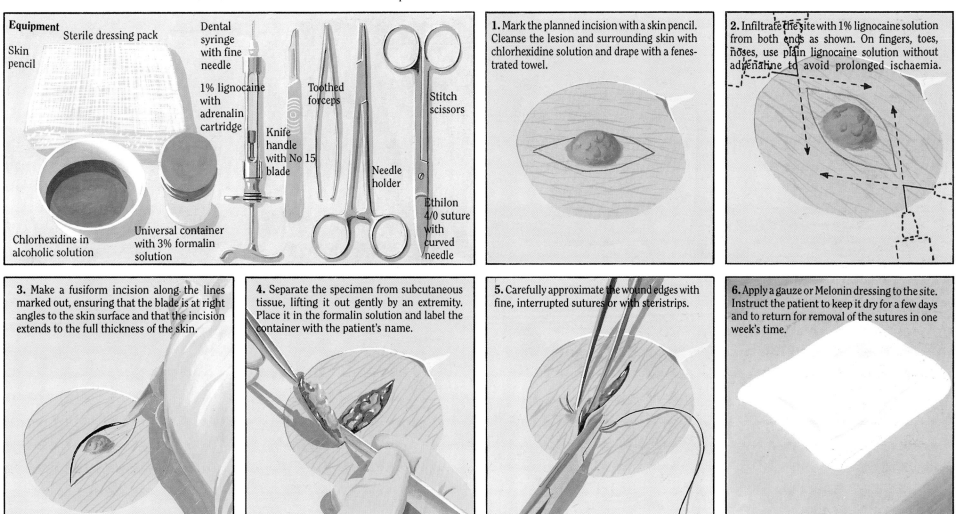

Equipment

Sterile dressing pack

Skin pencil

Dental syringe with fine needle

1% lignocaine with adrenalin cartridge

Knife handle with No 15 blade

Toothed forceps

Stitch scissors

Needle holder

Ethilon 4/0 suture with curved needle

Chlorhexidine in alcoholic solution

Universal container with 3% formalin solution

1. Mark the planned incision with a skin pencil. Cleanse the lesion and surrounding skin with chlorhexidine solution and drape with a fenestrated towel.

2. Infiltrate the site with 1% lignocaine solution from both ends as shown. On fingers, toes, noses, use plain lignocaine solution without adrenaline to avoid prolonged ischaemia.

3. Make a fusiform incision along the lines marked out, ensuring that the blade is at right angles to the skin surface and that the incision extends to the full thickness of the skin.

4. Separate the specimen from subcutaneous tissue, lifting it out gently by an extremity. Place it in the formalin solution and label the container with the patient's name.

5. Carefully approximate the wound edges with fine, interrupted sutures or with steristrips.

6. Apply a gauze or Melonin dressing to the site. Instruct the patient to keep it dry for a few days and to return for removal of the sutures in one week's time.

Fig. 7.31. Tumours: dermatofibroma.

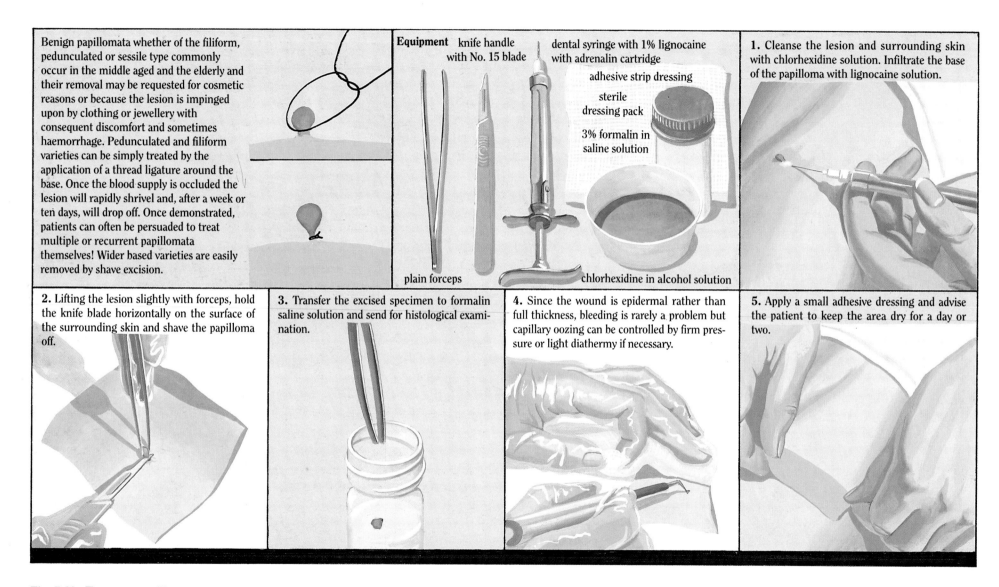

Benign papillomata whether of the filiform, pedunculated or sessile type commonly occur in the middle aged and the elderly and their removal may be requested for cosmetic reasons or because the lesion is impinged upon by clothing or jewellery with consequent discomfort and sometimes haemorrhage. Pedunculated and filiform varieties can be simply treated by the application of a thread ligature around the base. Once the blood supply is occluded the lesion will rapidly shrivel and, after a week or ten days, will drop off. Once demonstrated, patients can often be persuaded to treat multiple or recurrent papillomata themselves! Wider based varieties are easily removed by shave excision.

Equipment   knife handle with No. 15 blade   dental syringe with 1% lignocaine with adrenalin cartridge

adhesive strip dressing

sterile dressing pack

3% formalin in saline solution

plain forceps   chlorhexidine in alcohol solution

1. Cleanse the lesion and surrounding skin with chlorhexidine solution. Infiltrate the base of the papilloma with lignocaine solution.

2. Lifting the lesion slightly with forceps, hold the knife blade horizontally on the surface of the surrounding skin and shave the papilloma off.

3. Transfer the excised specimen to formalin saline solution and send for histological examination.

4. Since the wound is epidermal rather than full thickness, bleeding is rarely a problem but capillary oozing can be controlled by firm pressure or light diathermy if necessary.

5. Apply a small adhesive dressing and advise the patient to keep the area dry for a day or two.

Fig. 7.32. Tumours: papillomata.

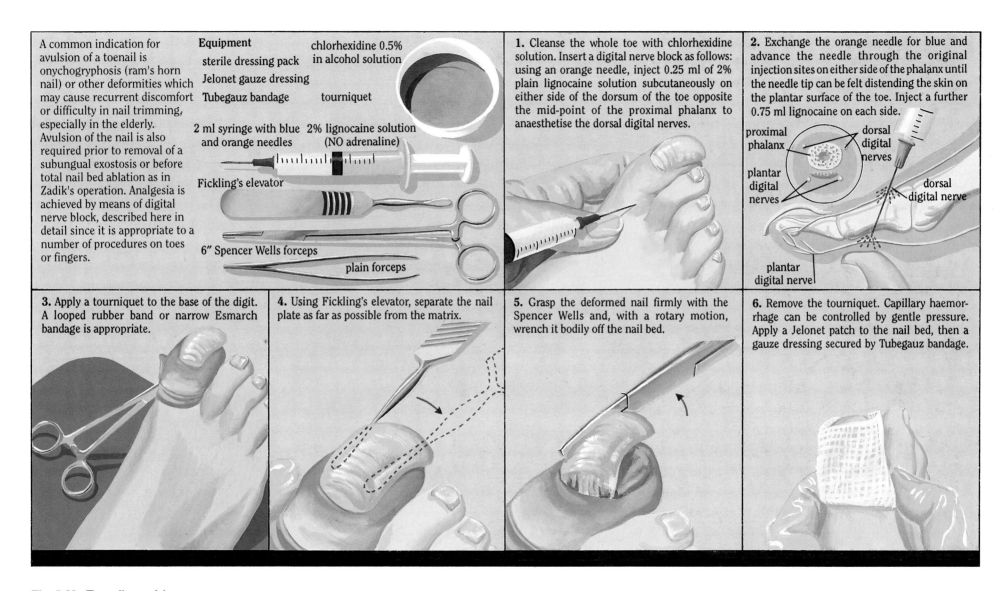

A common indication for avulsion of a toenail is onychogryphosis (ram's horn nail) or other deformities which may cause recurrent discomfort or difficulty in nail trimming, especially in the elderly. Avulsion of the nail is also required prior to removal of a subungual exostosis or before total nail bed ablation as in Zadik's operation. Analgesia is achieved by means of digital nerve block, described here in detail since it is appropriate to a number of procedures on toes or fingers.

Equipment
sterile dressing pack
Jelonet gauze dressing
Tubegauz bandage

chlorhexidine 0.5% in alcohol solution

tourniquet

2 ml syringe with blue and orange needles

2% lignocaine solution (NO adrenaline)

Fickling's elevator

6" Spencer Wells forceps

plain forceps

1. Cleanse the whole toe with chlorhexidine solution. Insert a digital nerve block as follows: using an orange needle, inject 0.25 ml of 2% plain lignocaine solution subcutaneously on either side of the dorsum of the toe opposite the mid-point of the proximal phalanx to anaesthetise the dorsal digital nerves.

2. Exchange the orange needle for blue and advance the needle through the original injection sites on either side of the phalanx until the needle tip can be felt distending the skin on the plantar surface of the toe. Inject a further 0.75 ml lignocaine on each side.

proximal phalanx

dorsal digital nerves

plantar digital nerves

dorsal digital nerve

plantar digital nerve

3. Apply a tourniquet to the base of the digit. A looped rubber band or narrow Esmarch bandage is appropriate.

4. Using Fickling's elevator, separate the nail plate as far as possible from the matrix.

5. Grasp the deformed nail firmly with the Spencer Wells and, with a rotary motion, wrench it bodily off the nail bed.

6. Remove the tourniquet. Capillary haemorrhage can be controlled by gentle pressure. Apply a Jelonet patch to the nail bed, then a gauze dressing secured by Tubegauz bandage.

Fig. 7.33. Toenails: avulsion.

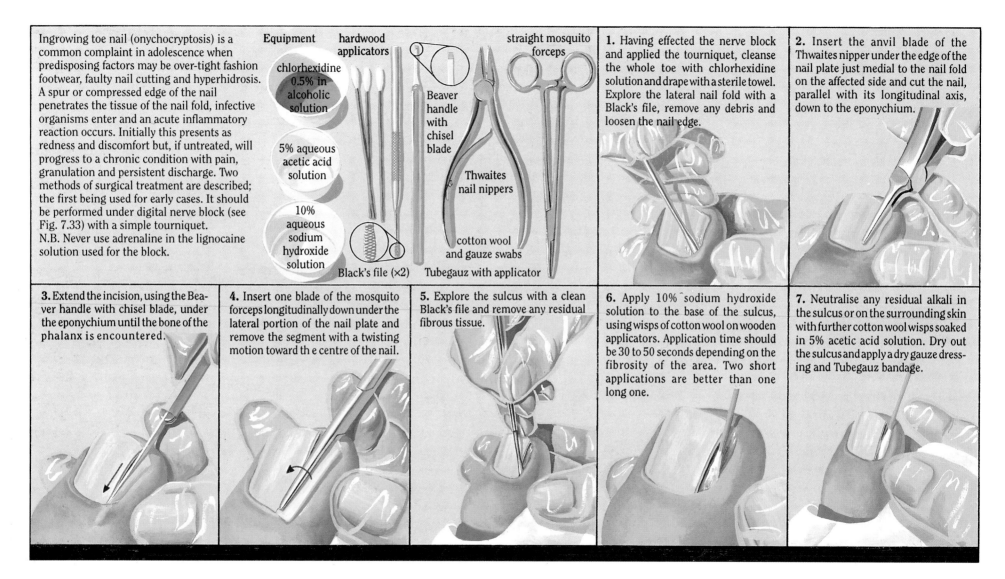

Ingrowing toe nail (onychocryptosis) is a common complaint in adolescence when predisposing factors may be over-tight fashion footwear, faulty nail cutting and hyperhidrosis. A spur or compressed edge of the nail penetrates the tissue of the nail fold, infective organisms enter and an acute inflammatory reaction occurs. Initially this presents as redness and discomfort but, if untreated, will progress to a chronic condition with pain, granulation and persistent discharge. Two methods of surgical treatment are described; the first being used for early cases. It should be performed under digital nerve block (see Fig. 7.33) with a simple tourniquet.
N.B. Never use adrenaline in the lignocaine solution used for the block.

Equipment

chlorhexidine 0.5% in alcoholic solution

5% aqueous acetic acid solution

10% aqueous sodium hydroxide solution

Black's file (×2)

hardwood applicators

Beaver handle with chisel blade

Thwaites nail nippers

straight mosquito forceps

cotton wool and gauze swabs

Tubegauz with applicator

1. Having effected the nerve block and applied the tourniquet, cleanse the whole toe with chlorhexidine solution and drape with a sterile towel. Explore the lateral nail fold with a Black's file, remove any debris and loosen the nail edge.

2. Insert the anvil blade of the Thwaites nipper under the edge of the nail plate just medial to the nail fold on the affected side and cut the nail, parallel with its longitudinal axis, down to the eponychium.

3. Extend the incision, using the Beaver handle with chisel blade, under the eponychium until the bone of the phalanx is encountered.

4. Insert one blade of the mosquito forceps longitudinally down under the lateral portion of the nail plate and remove the segment with a twisting motion toward the centre of the nail.

5. Explore the sulcus with a clean Black's file and remove any residual fibrous tissue.

6. Apply 10% sodium hydroxide solution to the base of the sulcus, using wisps of cotton wool on wooden applicators. Application time should be 30 to 50 seconds depending on the fibrosity of the area. Two short applications are better than one long one.

7. Neutralise any residual alkali in the sulcus or on the surrounding skin with further cotton wool wisps soaked in 5% acetic acid solution. Dry out the sulcus and apply a dry gauze dressing and Tubegauz bandage.

Fig. 7.34. Toenails: wedge resection (chiropody method).

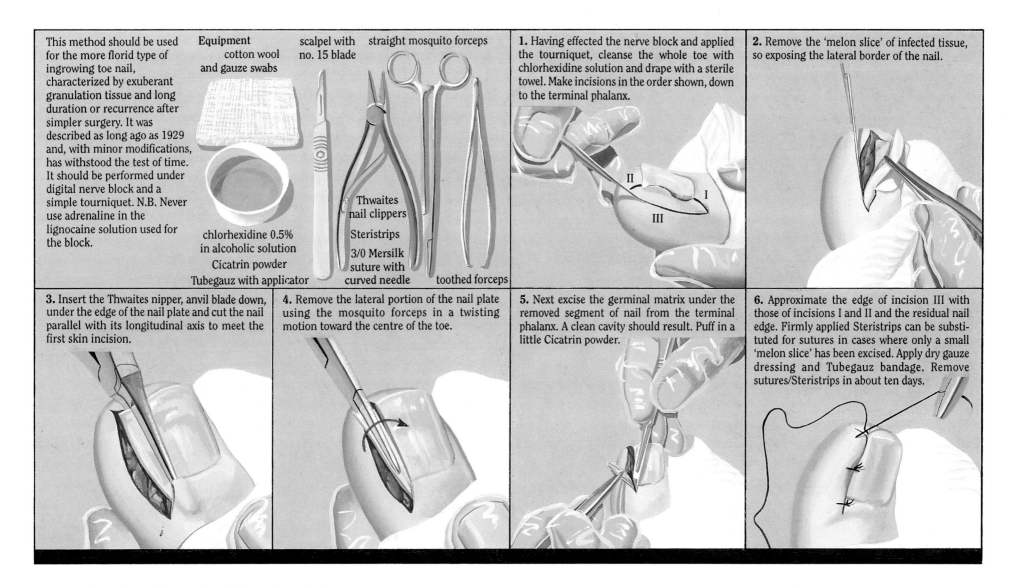

This method should be used for the more florid type of ingrowing toe nail, characterized by exuberant granulation tissue and long duration or recurrence after simpler surgery. It was described as long ago as 1929 and, with minor modifications, has withstood the test of time. It should be performed under digital nerve block and a simple tourniquet. N.B. Never use adrenaline in the lignocaine solution used for the block.

Equipment
cotton wool and gauze swabs

chlorhexidine 0.5% in alcoholic solution

Cicatrin powder

Tubegauz with applicator

scalpel with no. 15 blade

straight mosquito forceps

Thwaites nail clippers

Steristrips

3/0 Mersilk suture with curved needle

toothed forceps

1. Having effected the nerve block and applied the tourniquet, cleanse the whole toe with chlorhexidine solution and drape with a sterile towel. Make incisions in the order shown, down to the terminal phalanx.

2. Remove the 'melon slice' of infected tissue, so exposing the lateral border of the nail.

3. Insert the Thwaites nipper, anvil blade down, under the edge of the nail plate and cut the nail parallel with its longitudinal axis to meet the first skin incision.

4. Remove the lateral portion of the nail plate using the mosquito forceps in a twisting motion toward the centre of the toe.

5. Next excise the germinal matrix under the removed segment of nail from the terminal phalanx. A clean cavity should result. Puff in a little Cicatrin powder.

6. Approximate the edge of incision III with those of incisions I and II and the residual nail edge. Firmly applied Steristrips can be substituted for sutures in cases where only a small 'melon slice' has been excised. Apply dry gauze dressing and Tubegauz bandage. Remove sutures/Steristrips in about ten days.

Fig. 7.35. Toenails: wedge resection (Winograd method).

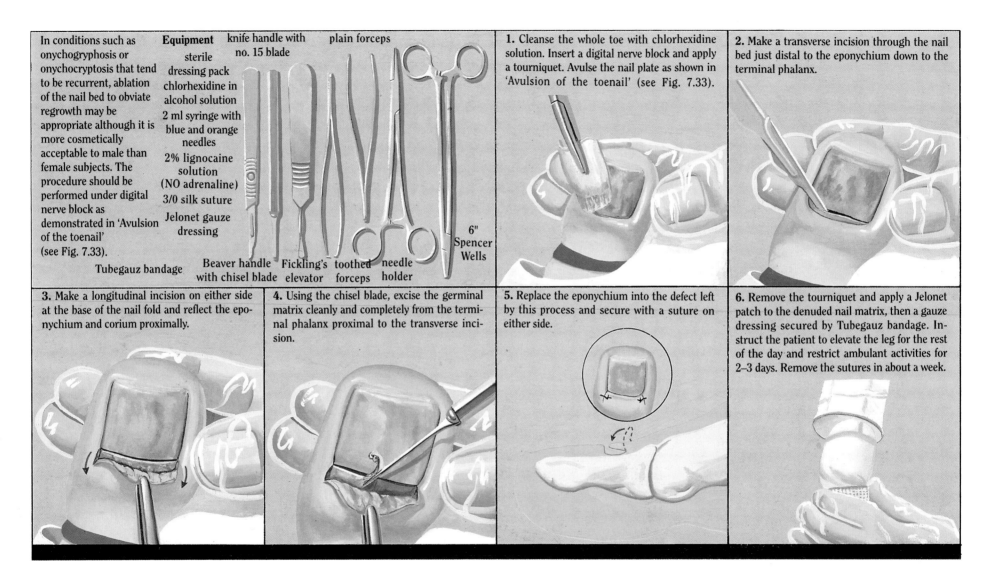

In conditions such as onychogryphosis or onychocryptosis that tend to be recurrent, ablation of the nail bed to obviate regrowth may be appropriate although it is more cosmetically acceptable to male than female subjects. The procedure should be performed under digital nerve block as demonstrated in 'Avulsion of the toenail' (see Fig. 7.33).

Equipment
sterile dressing pack
chlorhexidine in alcohol solution
2 ml syringe with blue and orange needles
2% lignocaine solution (NO adrenaline)
3/0 silk suture
Jelonet gauze dressing
Tubegauz bandage

knife handle with no. 15 blade

plain forceps

Beaver handle with chisel blade   Fickling's elevator   toothed forceps   needle holder   6" Spencer Wells

1. Cleanse the whole toe with chlorhexidine solution. Insert a digital nerve block and apply a tourniquet. Avulse the nail plate as shown in 'Avulsion of the toenail' (see Fig. 7.33).

2. Make a transverse incision through the nail bed just distal to the eponychium down to the terminal phalanx.

3. Make a longitudinal incision on either side at the base of the nail fold and reflect the eponychium and corium proximally.

4. Using the chisel blade, excise the germinal matrix cleanly and completely from the terminal phalanx proximal to the transverse incision.

5. Replace the eponychium into the defect left by this process and secure with a suture on either side.

6. Remove the tourniquet and apply a Jelonet patch to the denuded nail matrix, then a gauze dressing secured by Tubegauz bandage. Instruct the patient to elevate the leg for the rest of the day and restrict ambulant activities for 2–3 days. Remove the sutures in about a week.

Fig. 7.36. Toenails: ablation (Zadik method).

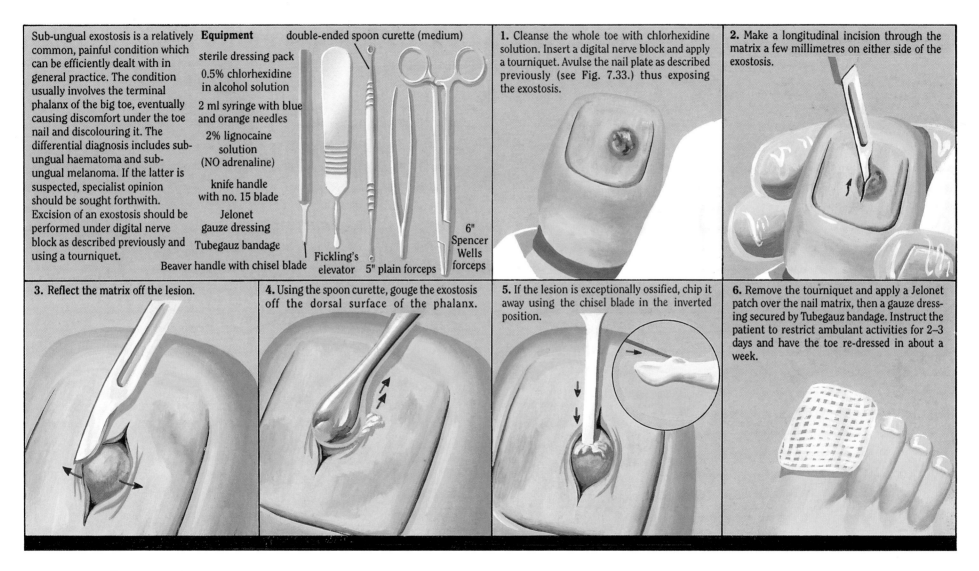

Sub-ungual exostosis is a relatively common, painful condition which can be efficiently dealt with in general practice. The condition usually involves the terminal phalanx of the big toe, eventually causing discomfort under the toe nail and discolouring it. The differential diagnosis includes sub-ungual haematoma and sub-ungual melanoma. If the latter is suspected, specialist opinion should be sought forthwith. Excision of an exostosis should be performed under digital nerve block as described previously and using a tourniquet.

Equipment

sterile dressing pack

0.5% chlorhexidine in alcohol solution

2 ml syringe with blue and orange needles

2% lignocaine solution (NO adrenaline)

knife handle with no. 15 blade

Jelonet gauze dressing

Tubegauz bandage

Beaver handle with chisel blade

double-ended spoon curette (medium)

Fickling's elevator

5" plain forceps

6" Spencer Wells forceps

1. Cleanse the whole toe with chlorhexidine solution. Insert a digital nerve block and apply a tourniquet. Avulse the nail plate as described previously (see Fig. 7.33.) thus exposing the exostosis.

2. Make a longitudinal incision through the matrix a few millimetres on either side of the exostosis.

3. Reflect the matrix off the lesion.

4. Using the spoon curette, gouge the exostosis off the dorsal surface of the phalanx.

5. If the lesion is exceptionally ossified, chip it away using the chisel blade in the inverted position.

6. Remove the tourniquet and apply a Jelonet patch over the nail matrix, then a gauze dressing secured by Tubegauz bandage. Instruct the patient to restrict ambulant activities for 2–3 days and have the toe re-dressed in about a week.

Fig. 7.37. Toenails: subungual exostosis.

Skin conditions often occur in multivariate and atypical forms so that clinical diagnosis is not always possible with accuracy. In such cases, precise diagnosis may be achieved by histological examination of a small section of the lesion, that is, a biopsy. Small lesions (say, not more than 1.5cm in diameter) should be excised completely taking care to preserve a narrow surround of normal tissue. Larger lesions may be biopsied either radially or tangentially, again including a small area of normal tissue on the periphery. Specimens should be transferred to the laboratory in 3% formalin in normal saline solution with full clinical details.

Equipment

sterile dressing pack
chlorhexidine in alcohol solution
dental syringe with fine needle
and 1% lignocaine with adrenalin cartridge
knife handle with No. 11 blade
plain forceps
toothed forceps
needle holder
Ethilon 4/0 suture with curved needle
stitch scissors
universal container with formalin solution

1. Cleanse the lesion and surrounding skin with chlorhexidine solution. Infiltrate the biopsy site with lignocaine solution. On fingers, toes, noses, use plain solution **without** adrenalin.

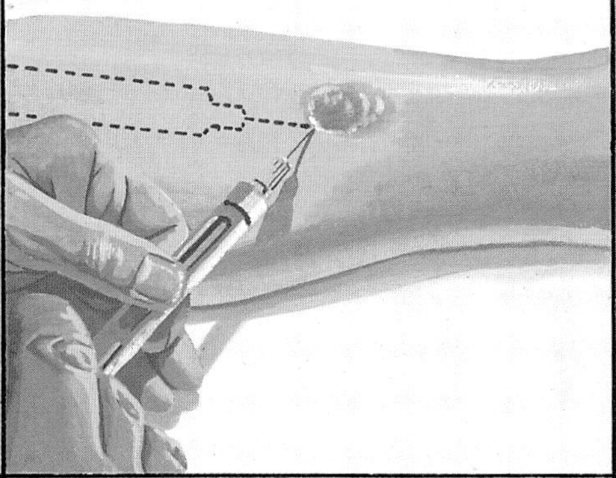

2. Make an elliptical incision about 1.0 by 0.5cm aligned with skin creases, if any. Ensure that the blade is held at right angles to the skin surface and extends full thickness and that a small area of normal tissue is included.

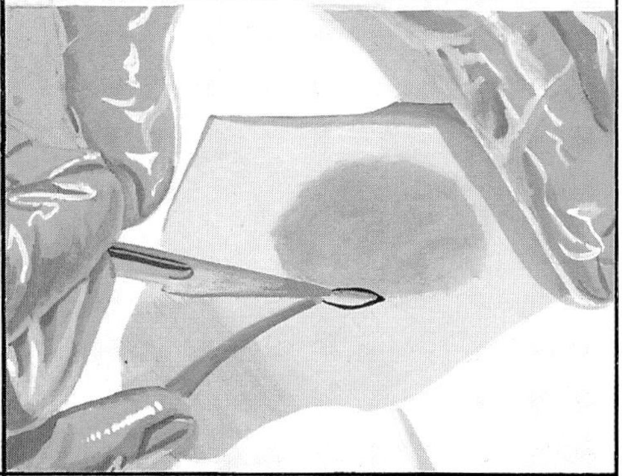

3. Separate the specimen from subcutaneous tissue; lift out gently with plain forceps and place it in the formalin solution. Don't forget to label the container.

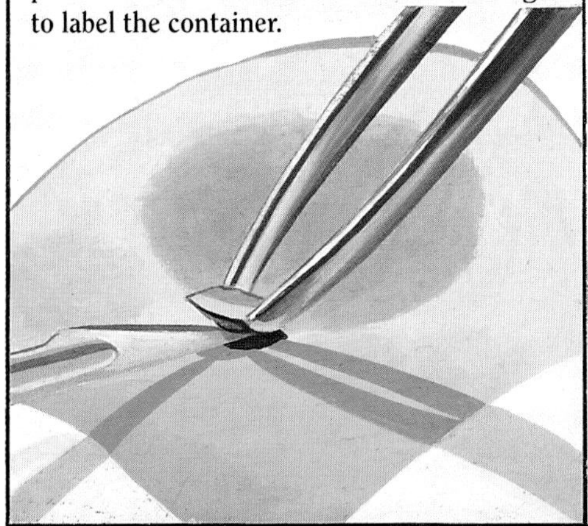

4. Dry out the wound with a gauze swab and ensure that no major bleeding points persist.

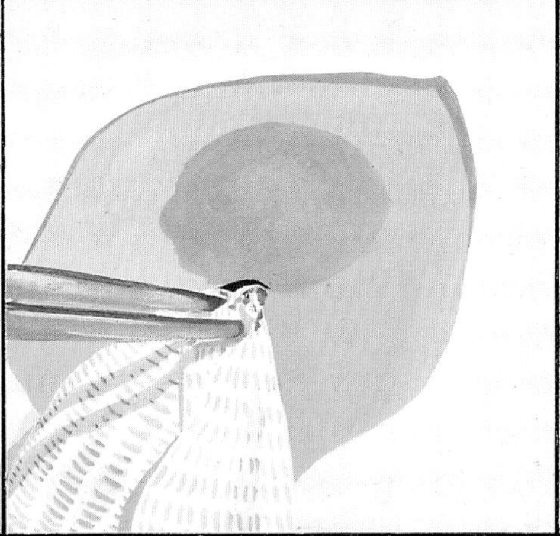

5. Suture the wound with two or three interrupted Ethilon sutures.

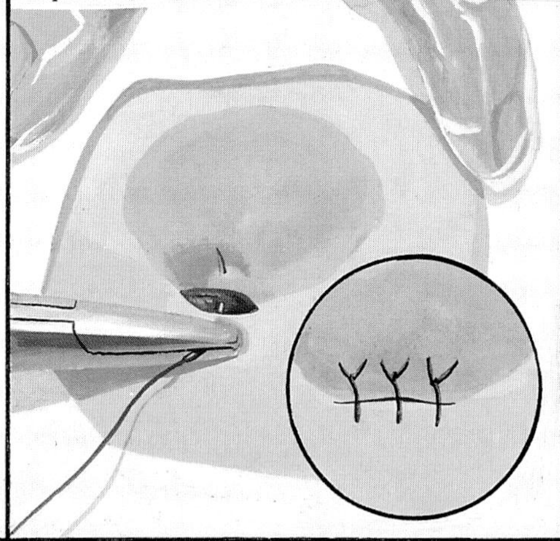

6. Apply a gauze or Melolin dressing. Instruct the patient to keep the site dry for a few days and return for removal of sutures in one week.

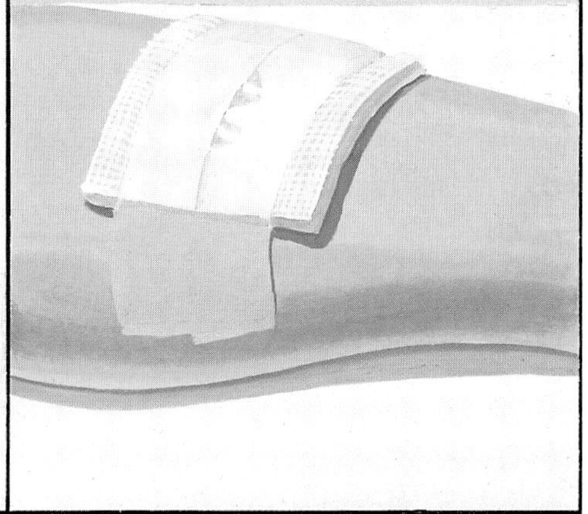

Fig. 7.38. Other dermatological: excision biopsy.

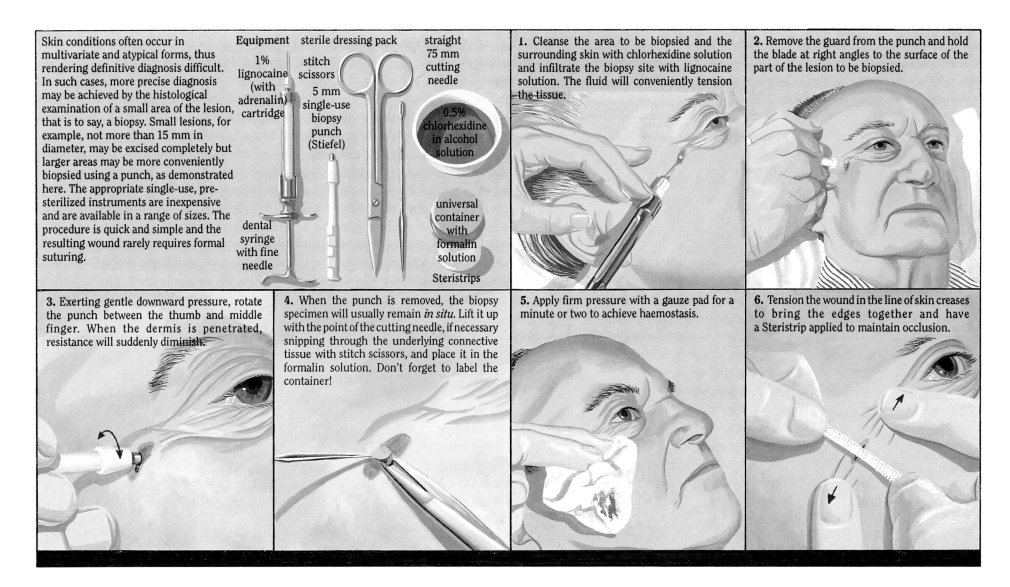

Skin conditions often occur in multivariate and atypical forms, thus rendering definitive diagnosis difficult. In such cases, more precise diagnosis may be achieved by the histological examination of a small area of the lesion, that is to say, a biopsy. Small lesions, for example, not more than 15 mm in diameter, may be excised completely but larger areas may be more conveniently biopsied using a punch, as demonstrated here. The appropriate single-use, pre-sterilized instruments are inexpensive and are available in a range of sizes. The procedure is quick and simple and the resulting wound rarely requires formal suturing.

Equipment   sterile dressing pack   straight 75 mm cutting needle

1% lignocaine (with adrenalin) cartridge

stitch scissors

5 mm single-use biopsy punch (Stiefel)

0.5% chlorhexidine in alcohol solution

universal container with formalin solution

Steristrips

dental syringe with fine needle

1. Cleanse the area to be biopsied and the surrounding skin with chlorhexidine solution and infiltrate the biopsy site with lignocaine solution. The fluid will conveniently tension the tissue.

2. Remove the guard from the punch and hold the blade at right angles to the surface of the part of the lesion to be biopsied.

3. Exerting gentle downward pressure, rotate the punch between the thumb and middle finger. When the dermis is penetrated, resistance will suddenly diminish.

4. When the punch is removed, the biopsy specimen will usually remain *in situ*. Lift it up with the point of the cutting needle, if necessary snipping through the underlying connective tissue with stitch scissors, and place it in the formalin solution. Don't forget to label the container!

5. Apply firm pressure with a gauze pad for a minute or two to achieve haemostasis.

6. Tension the wound in the line of skin creases to bring the edges together and have a Steristrip applied to maintain occlusion.

Fig. 7.39. Other dermatological: shave and punch biopsy.

Curette, cautery, and cryosurgery

Introduction

The techniques of curettage, cautery, and cryotherapy readily lend themselves to the management of a wide variety of common dermatological conditions and the equipment required need not be especially expensive. However, these methods are necessarily destructive so, before employing them, the practitioner must be in no doubt as to the nature of the lesion concerned and, in particular, that it is of a benign character. Should uncertainty exist, then it must be excised, as described earlier on page 32 and sent for histological examination.

Apart from warts and verrucae, the treatment of 'other skin lesions' such as molluscum contagiosum, is allowable in this category. Since the treatment of molluscum contagiosum is traditionally by means of chemotherapy one wonders whether chemical cautery of other conditions such as peri-anal condylomata or even the ablation of granulation tissue with silver nitrate would also be approved? In this context, the advice of individual FHSA medical advisors should be sought before submitting claims for payment.

Further reading

Cracknell, I. and Mead, M. (1991). Electrocautery and cryocautery. *Update*, **42**, 118–4.

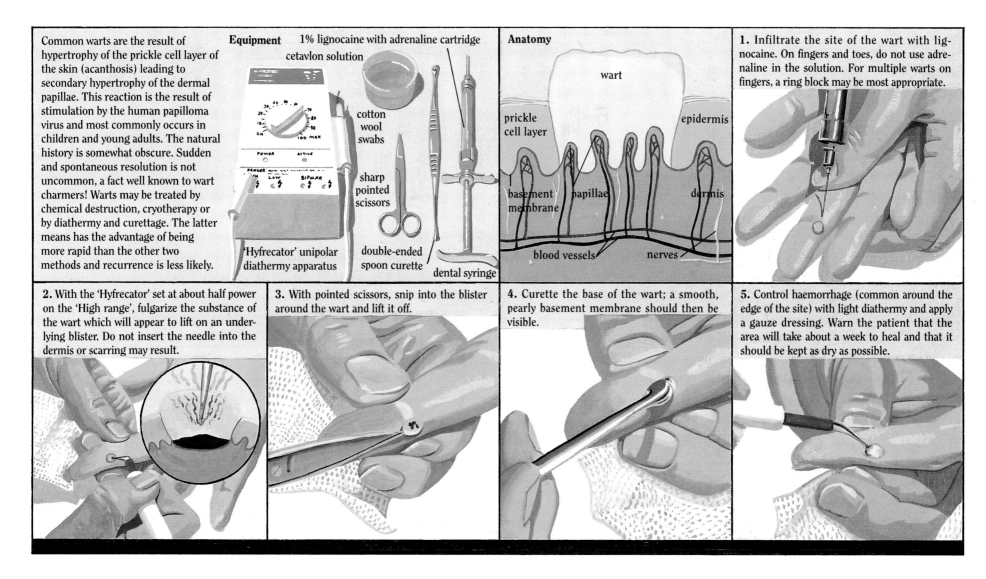

Common warts are the result of hypertrophy of the prickle cell layer of the skin (acanthosis) leading to secondary hypertrophy of the dermal papillae. This reaction is the result of stimulation by the human papilloma virus and most commonly occurs in children and young adults. The natural history is somewhat obscure. Sudden and spontaneous resolution is not uncommon, a fact well known to wart charmers! Warts may be treated by chemical destruction, cryotherapy or by diathermy and curettage. The latter means has the advantage of being more rapid than the other two methods and recurrence is less likely.

Equipment 1% lignocaine with adrenaline cartridge
cetavlon solution
cotton wool swabs
sharp pointed scissors
'Hyfrecator' unipolar diathermy apparatus
double-ended spoon curette
dental syringe

Anatomy
wart
prickle cell layer
epidermis
basement membrane
papillae
dermis
blood vessels
nerves

1. Infiltrate the site of the wart with lignocaine. On fingers and toes, do not use adrenaline in the solution. For multiple warts on fingers, a ring block may be most appropriate.

2. With the 'Hyfrecator' set at about half power on the 'High range', fulgarize the substance of the wart which will appear to lift on an underlying blister. Do not insert the needle into the dermis or scarring may result.

3. With pointed scissors, snip into the blister around the wart and lift it off.

4. Curette the base of the wart; a smooth, pearly basement membrane should then be visible.

5. Control haemorrhage (common around the edge of the site) with light diathermy and apply a gauze dressing. Warn the patient that the area will take about a week to heal and that it should be kept as dry as possible.

Fig. 7.40. Common warts: diathermy.

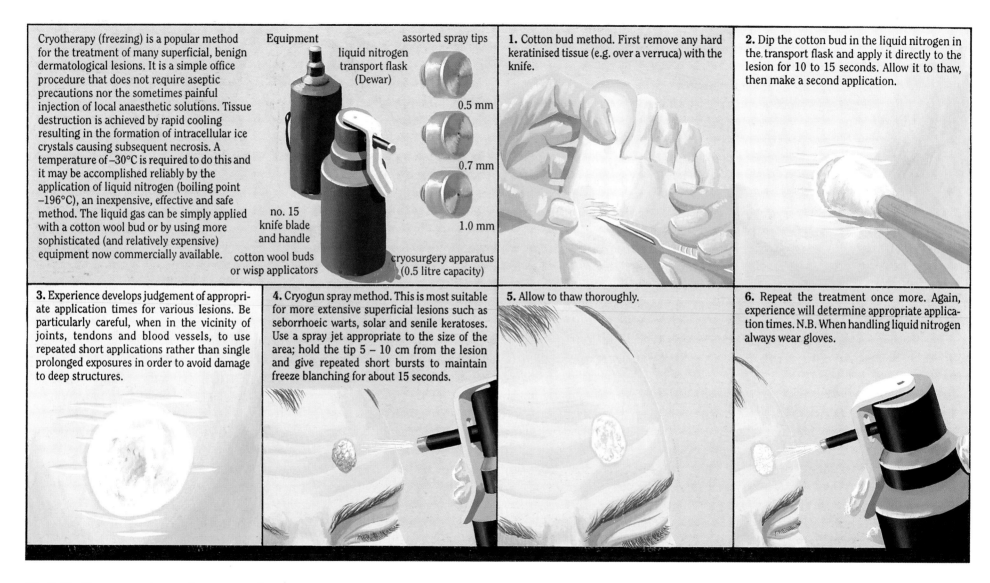

Cryotherapy (freezing) is a popular method for the treatment of many superficial, benign dermatological lesions. It is a simple office procedure that does not require aseptic precautions nor the sometimes painful injection of local anaesthetic solutions. Tissue destruction is achieved by rapid cooling resulting in the formation of intracellular ice crystals causing subsequent necrosis. A temperature of −30°C is required to do this and it may be accomplished reliably by the application of liquid nitrogen (boiling point −196°C), an inexpensive, effective and safe method. The liquid gas can be simply applied with a cotton wool bud or by using more sophisticated (and relatively expensive) equipment now commercially available.

Equipment

liquid nitrogen transport flask (Dewar)

assorted spray tips

0.5 mm

0.7 mm

1.0 mm

no. 15 knife blade and handle

cotton wool buds or wisp applicators

cryosurgery apparatus (0.5 litre capacity)

1. Cotton bud method. First remove any hard keratinised tissue (e.g. over a verruca) with the knife.

2. Dip the cotton bud in the liquid nitrogen in the transport flask and apply it directly to the lesion for 10 to 15 seconds. Allow it to thaw, then make a second application.

3. Experience develops judgement of appropriate application times for various lesions. Be particularly careful, when in the vicinity of joints, tendons and blood vessels, to use repeated short applications rather than single prolonged exposures in order to avoid damage to deep structures.

4. Cryogun spray method. This is most suitable for more extensive superficial lesions such as seborrhoeic warts, solar and senile keratoses. Use a spray jet appropriate to the size of the area; hold the tip 5 – 10 cm from the lesion and give repeated short bursts to maintain freeze blanching for about 15 seconds.

5. Allow to thaw thoroughly.

6. Repeat the treatment once more. Again, experience will determine appropriate application times. N.B. When handling liquid nitrogen always wear gloves.

Fig. 7.41. Common warts: cryotherapy, part I.

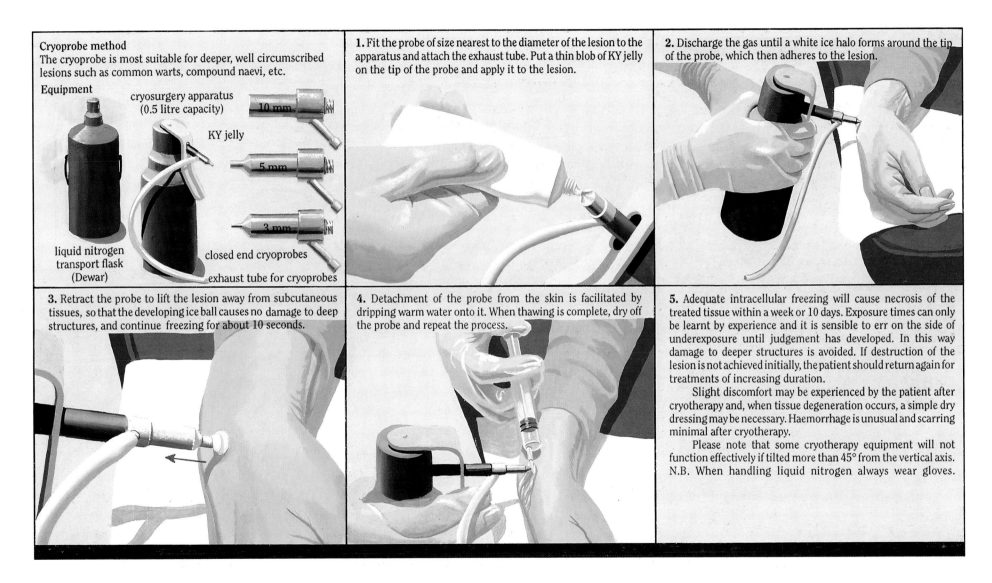

Cryoprobe method
The cryoprobe is most suitable for deeper, well circumscribed lesions such as common warts, compound naevi, etc.

Equipment
cryosurgery apparatus (0.5 litre capacity)
KY jelly
10 mm
5 mm
3 mm
liquid nitrogen transport flask (Dewar)
closed end cryoprobes
exhaust tube for cryoprobes

1. Fit the probe of size nearest to the diameter of the lesion to the apparatus and attach the exhaust tube. Put a thin blob of KY jelly on the tip of the probe and apply it to the lesion.

2. Discharge the gas until a white ice halo forms around the tip of the probe, which then adheres to the lesion.

3. Retract the probe to lift the lesion away from subcutaneous tissues, so that the developing ice ball causes no damage to deep structures, and continue freezing for about 10 seconds.

4. Detachment of the probe from the skin is facilitated by dripping warm water onto it. When thawing is complete, dry off the probe and repeat the process.

5. Adequate intracellular freezing will cause necrosis of the treated tissue within a week or 10 days. Exposure times can only be learnt by experience and it is sensible to err on the side of underexposure until judgement has developed. In this way damage to deeper structures is avoided. If destruction of the lesion is not achieved initially, the patient should return again for treatments of increasing duration.

Slight discomfort may be experienced by the patient after cryotherapy and, when tissue degeneration occurs, a simple dry dressing may be necessary. Haemorrhage is unusual and scarring minimal after cryotherapy.

Please note that some cryotherapy equipment will not function effectively if tilted more than 45° from the vertical axis. N.B. When handling liquid nitrogen always wear gloves.

Fig. 7.42. Common warts: cryotherapy, part II.

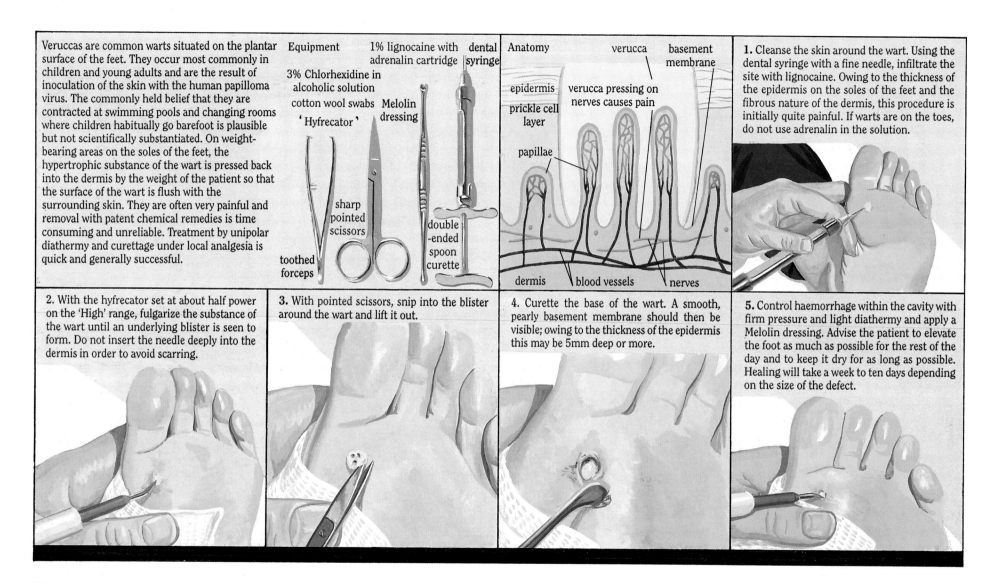

Veruccas are common warts situated on the plantar surface of the feet. They occur most commonly in children and young adults and are the result of inoculation of the skin with the human papilloma virus. The commonly held belief that they are contracted at swimming pools and changing rooms where children habitually go barefoot is plausible but not scientifically substantiated. On weight-bearing areas on the soles of the feet, the hypertrophic substance of the wart is pressed back into the dermis by the weight of the patient so that the surface of the wart is flush with the surrounding skin. They are often very painful and removal with patent chemical remedies is time consuming and unreliable. Treatment by unipolar diathermy and curettage under local analgesia is quick and generally successful.

Equipment   1% lignocaine with   dental
adrenalin cartridge   syringe
3% Chlorhexidine in alcoholic solution
cotton wool swabs   Melolin dressing
' Hyfrecator '
toothed forceps   sharp pointed scissors   double-ended spoon curette

Anatomy   verucca   basement membrane
epidermis   verucca pressing on nerves causes pain
prickle cell layer
papillae
dermis   blood vessels   nerves

1. Cleanse the skin around the wart. Using the dental syringe with a fine needle, infiltrate the site with lignocaine. Owing to the thickness of the epidermis on the soles of the feet and the fibrous nature of the dermis, this procedure is initially quite painful. If warts are on the toes, do not use adrenalin in the solution.

2. With the hyfrecator set at about half power on the 'High' range, fulgarize the substance of the wart until an underlying blister is seen to form. Do not insert the needle deeply into the dermis in order to avoid scarring.

3. With pointed scissors, snip into the blister around the wart and lift it out.

4. Curette the base of the wart. A smooth, pearly basement membrane should then be visible; owing to the thickness of the epidermis this may be 5mm deep or more.

5. Control haemorrhage within the cavity with firm pressure and light diathermy and apply a Melolin dressing. Advise the patient to elevate the foot as much as possible for the rest of the day and to keep it dry for as long as possible. Healing will take a week to ten days depending on the size of the defect.

Fig. 7.43. Plantar warts: diathermy.

Condylomata acuminata, or genital warts, are exuberant papilliferous outgrowths occuring on and around the anal and vaginal orifices. This epithelial reaction is the result of stimulation by the human papilloma virus, which seems to thrive in the moist, warm environment of the perineum. Condylomata are often contracted through sexual activity and are more common in homosexual men. In women there appears to be an association of condylomata with subsequent dystrophic changes in the cervical epithelium. For this reason annual cytological examination should be performed until negative results have been obtained for five years. Genital warts may be treated by chemical destruction, cryotherapy or, in extreme cases, diathermy under general anaesthesia.

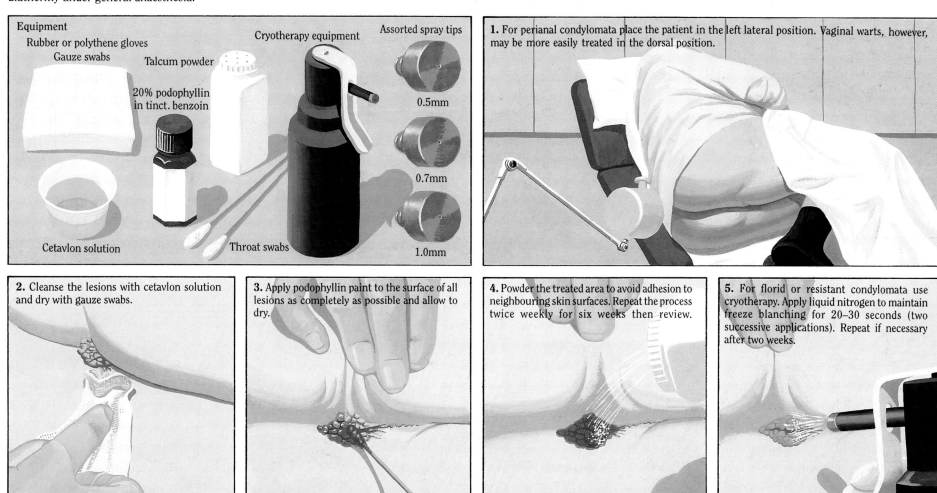

Equipment
Rubber or polythene gloves
Gauze swabs
Talcum powder
Cryotherapy equipment
Assorted spray tips
20% podophyllin in tinct. benzoin
0.5mm
0.7mm
Cetavlon solution
Throat swabs
1.0mm

1. For perianal condylomata place the patient in the left lateral position. Vaginal warts, however, may be more easily treated in the dorsal position.

2. Cleanse the lesions with cetavlon solution and dry with gauze swabs.

3. Apply podophyllin paint to the surface of all lesions as completely as possible and allow to dry.

4. Powder the treated area to avoid adhesion to neighbouring skin surfaces. Repeat the process twice weekly for six weeks then review.

5. For florid or resistant condylomata use cryotherapy. Apply liquid nitrogen to maintain freeze blanching for 20–30 seconds (two successive applications). Repeat if necessary after two weeks.

Fig. 7.44. Condylomata: chemotherapy and cryotherapy.

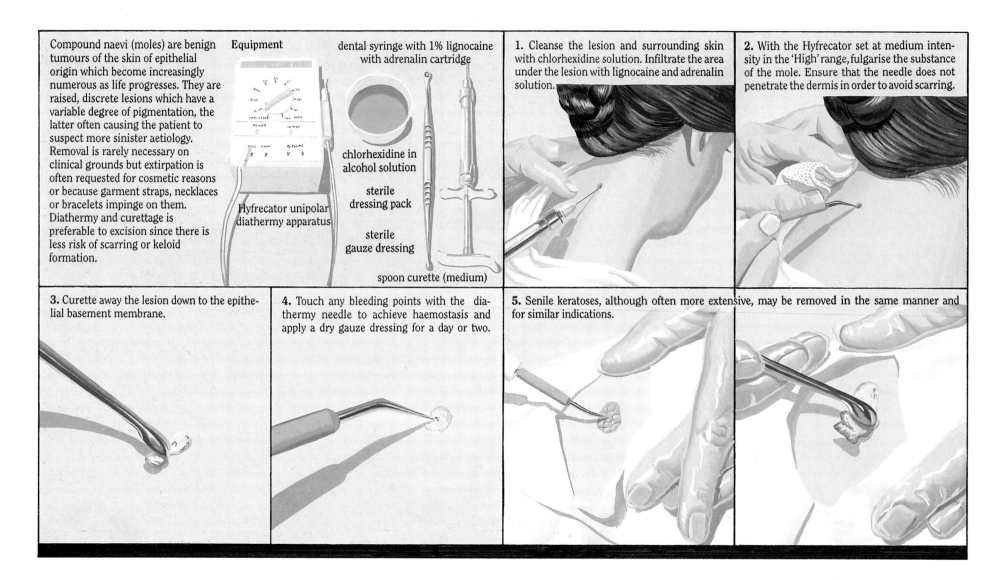

Compound naevi (moles) are benign tumours of the skin of epithelial origin which become increasingly numerous as life progresses. They are raised, discrete lesions which have a variable degree of pigmentation, the latter often causing the patient to suspect more sinister aetiology. Removal is rarely necessary on clinical grounds but extirpation is often requested for cosmetic reasons or because garment straps, necklaces or bracelets impinge on them. Diathermy and curettage is preferable to excision since there is less risk of scarring or keloid formation.

Equipment

Hyfrecator unipolar diathermy apparatus

dental syringe with 1% lignocaine with adrenalin cartridge

chlorhexidine in alcohol solution

sterile dressing pack

sterile gauze dressing

spoon curette (medium)

1. Cleanse the lesion and surrounding skin with chlorhexidine solution. Infiltrate the area under the lesion with lignocaine and adrenalin solution.

2. With the Hyfrecator set at medium intensity in the 'High' range, fulgarise the substance of the mole. Ensure that the needle does not penetrate the dermis in order to avoid scarring.

3. Curette away the lesion down to the epithelial basement membrane.

4. Touch any bleeding points with the diathermy needle to achieve haemostasis and apply a dry gauze dressing for a day or two.

5. Senile keratoses, although often more extensive, may be removed in the same manner and for similar indications.

Fig. 7.45. Compound naevi and senile keratoses: diathermy.

Spider naevi are typified by a central papule on the surface of the skin surrounded by feeder vessels. The central papule is a dilated venule. They are commonly found on the face, torso and limbs, in children as well as adults. If large numbers are present one should consider conditions such as hereditary harmorrhagic telangiectasia and liver failure. More commonly they are associated with pregnancy and the contraceptive pill.

Spider naevi tend to enlarge during pregnancy and are best left until a few months after the birth as they may regress spontaneously. The patient should return to the surgery 3–4 weeks after treatment and the procedure repeated if necessary.

Equipment

good light source

gloves

hyfrecator   fine needle (e.g. epilation needle)

1. Clean the area with an antiseptic agent. Avoid alcohol-based cleansing solutions because of high temperatures produced by the hyfrecator.

2. Infiltrate the skin around the naevus with plain lignocaine. Fan the anaesthetic if necessary.

3. Attach an epilation needle to the handle of the hyfrecator.

4. Switch on the hyfrecator and turn the dial to 30–50 in the low range.

5. Apply the needle into the central papule.

6. The area turns white upon application of the needle due to a combination of vessel obliteration and vasoconstriction. No dressing is necessary.

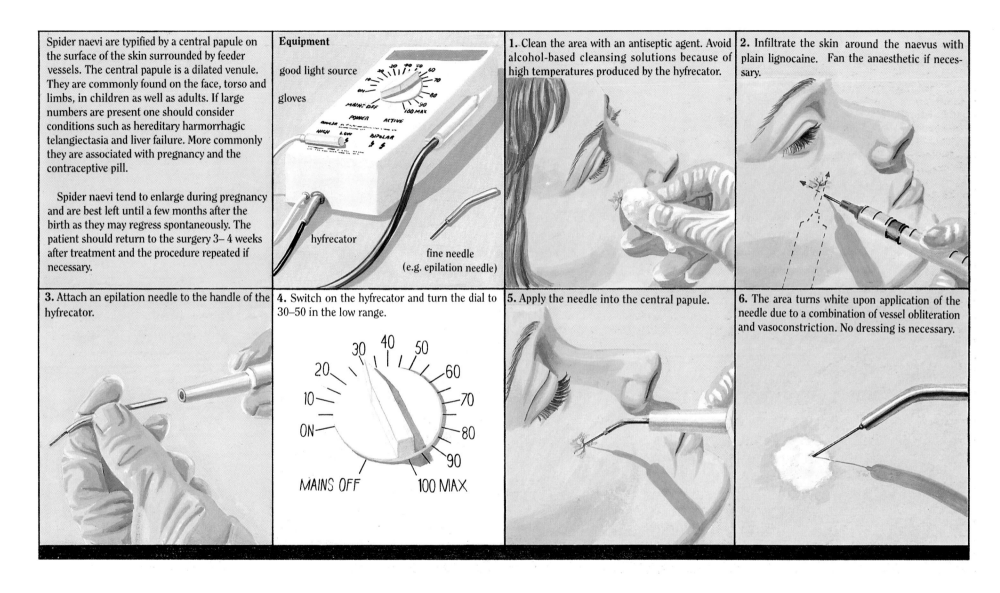

Fig. 7.46. Spider naevi and teleangiectasia.

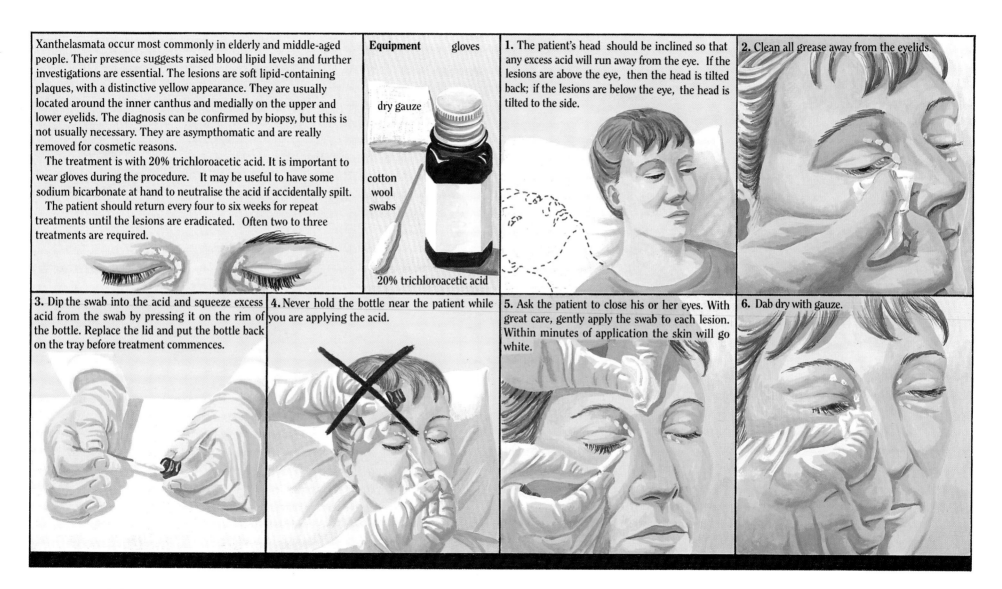

Xanthelasmata occur most commonly in elderly and middle-aged people. Their presence suggests raised blood lipid levels and further investigations are essential. The lesions are soft lipid-containing plaques, with a distinctive yellow appearance. They are usually located around the inner canthus and medially on the upper and lower eyelids. The diagnosis can be confirmed by biopsy, but this is not usually necessary. They are asympthomatic and are really removed for cosmetic reasons.

The treatment is with 20% trichloroacetic acid. It is important to wear gloves during the procedure. It may be useful to have some sodium bicarbonate at hand to neutralise the acid if accidentally spilt.

The patient should return every four to six weeks for repeat treatments until the lesions are eradicated. Often two to three treatments are required.

Equipment   gloves

dry gauze

cotton wool swabs

20% trichloroacetic acid

1. The patient's head should be inclined so that any excess acid will run away from the eye. If the lesions are above the eye, then the head is tilted back; if the lesions are below the eye, the head is tilted to the side.

2. Clean all grease away from the eyelids.

3. Dip the swab into the acid and squeeze excess acid from the swab by pressing it on the rim of the bottle. Replace the lid and put the bottle back on the tray before treatment commences.

4. Never hold the bottle near the patient while you are applying the acid.

5. Ask the patient to close his or her eyes. With great care, gently apply the swab to each lesion. Within minutes of application the skin will go white.

6. Dab dry with gauze.

Fig. 7.47. Xanthelasma.

Other procedures

Introduction

'Other' allowable minor surgical procedures under the New Contract might be expected to cover a wide spectrum of conditions, including the repair of lacerations, but, at the time of writing, this category appears only to include the removal of foreign bodies (from various orifices and from the skin) and nasal cautery for the control of epistaxis. Small children have a propensity for the experimental insertion of foreign bodies into natural orifices and, where access to hospital accident and emergency departments is not immediately available, the anxious parent will usually seek the assistance of their general practitioner. Satisfactory management of these situations is dependent on the availability of a calm and confident assistant who can correctly control the frightened subject whilst the doctor utilizes one or other of the simple tricks of the trade to recover the offending object.

In cases where the foreign body has penetrated the integument however, the doctor must make certain decisions before attempting its removal.

(1) Is the foreign body accurately localized?
(2) Are any vital subcutaneous structures involved?
(3) Can adequate analgesia be achieved?
(4) Is it feasible to obtain a bloodless operation field?

If the answers to these questions are less than satisfactory, the patient should be referred to a hospital casualty department.

Further reading
Kyle, J., Smith, J. A. R. and Johnston, D. (1992). *Pye's surgical handicraft* (22nd edn), p. 54. Butterworth-Heinemann, Oxford.

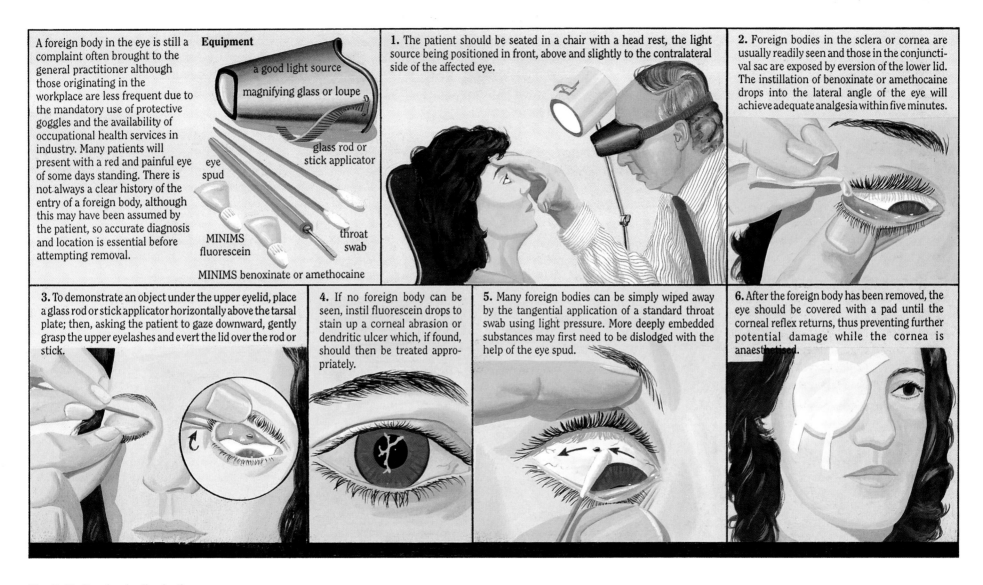

A foreign body in the eye is still a complaint often brought to the general practitioner although those originating in the workplace are less frequent due to the mandatory use of protective goggles and the availability of occupational health services in industry. Many patients will present with a red and painful eye of some days standing. There is not always a clear history of the entry of a foreign body, although this may have been assumed by the patient, so accurate diagnosis and location is essential before attempting removal.

Equipment

a good light source

magnifying glass or loupe

glass rod or stick applicator

eye spud

throat swab

MINIMS fluorescein

MINIMS benoxinate or amethocaine

1. The patient should be seated in a chair with a head rest, the light source being positioned in front, above and slightly to the contralateral side of the affected eye.

2. Foreign bodies in the sclera or cornea are usually readily seen and those in the conjunctival sac are exposed by eversion of the lower lid. The instillation of benoxinate or amethocaine drops into the lateral angle of the eye will achieve adequate analgesia within five minutes.

3. To demonstrate an object under the upper eyelid, place a glass rod or stick applicator horizontally above the tarsal plate; then, asking the patient to gaze downward, gently grasp the upper eyelashes and evert the lid over the rod or stick.

4. If no foreign body can be seen, instil fluorescein drops to stain up a corneal abrasion or dendritic ulcer which, if found, should then be treated appropriately.

5. Many foreign bodies can be simply wiped away by the tangential application of a standard throat swab using light pressure. More deeply embedded substances may first need to be dislodged with the help of the eye spud.

6. After the foreign body has been removed, the eye should be covered with a pad until the corneal reflex returns, thus preventing further potential damage while the cornea is anaesthetised.

Fig. 7.48. Foreign bodies in the eye.

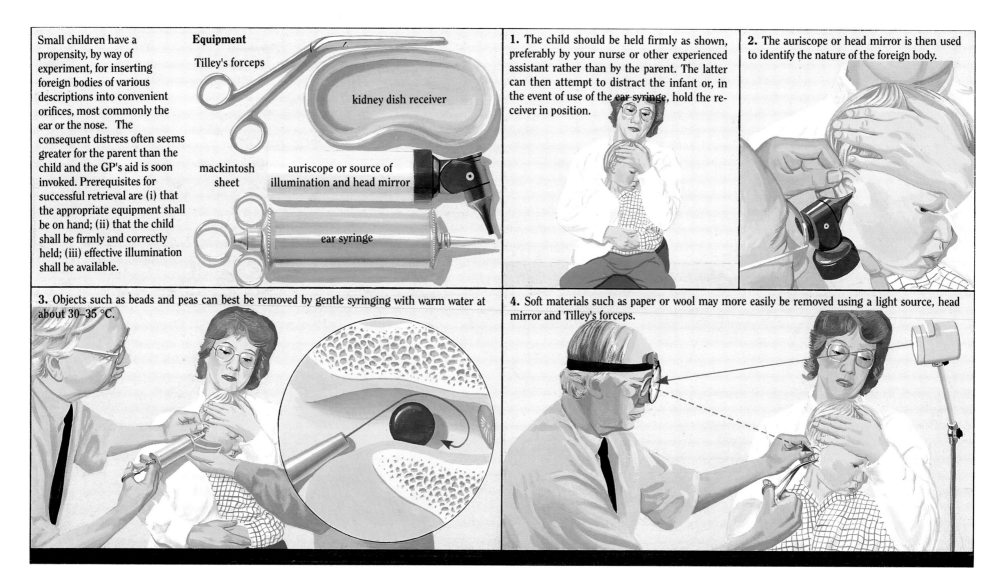

Small children have a propensity, by way of experiment, for inserting foreign bodies of various descriptions into convenient orifices, most commonly the ear or the nose. The consequent distress often seems greater for the parent than the child and the GP's aid is soon invoked. Prerequisites for successful retrieval are (i) that the appropriate equipment shall be on hand; (ii) that the child shall be firmly and correctly held; (iii) effective illumination shall be available.

Equipment

Tilley's forceps

kidney dish receiver

mackintosh sheet

auriscope or source of illumination and head mirror

ear syringe

1. The child should be held firmly as shown, preferably by your nurse or other experienced assistant rather than by the parent. The latter can then attempt to distract the infant or, in the event of use of the ear syringe, hold the receiver in position.

2. The auriscope or head mirror is then used to identify the nature of the foreign body.

3. Objects such as beads and peas can best be removed by gentle syringing with warm water at about 30–35 °C.

4. Soft materials such as paper or wool may more easily be removed using a light source, head mirror and Tilley's forceps.

Fig. 7.49. Foreign bodies in the ear.

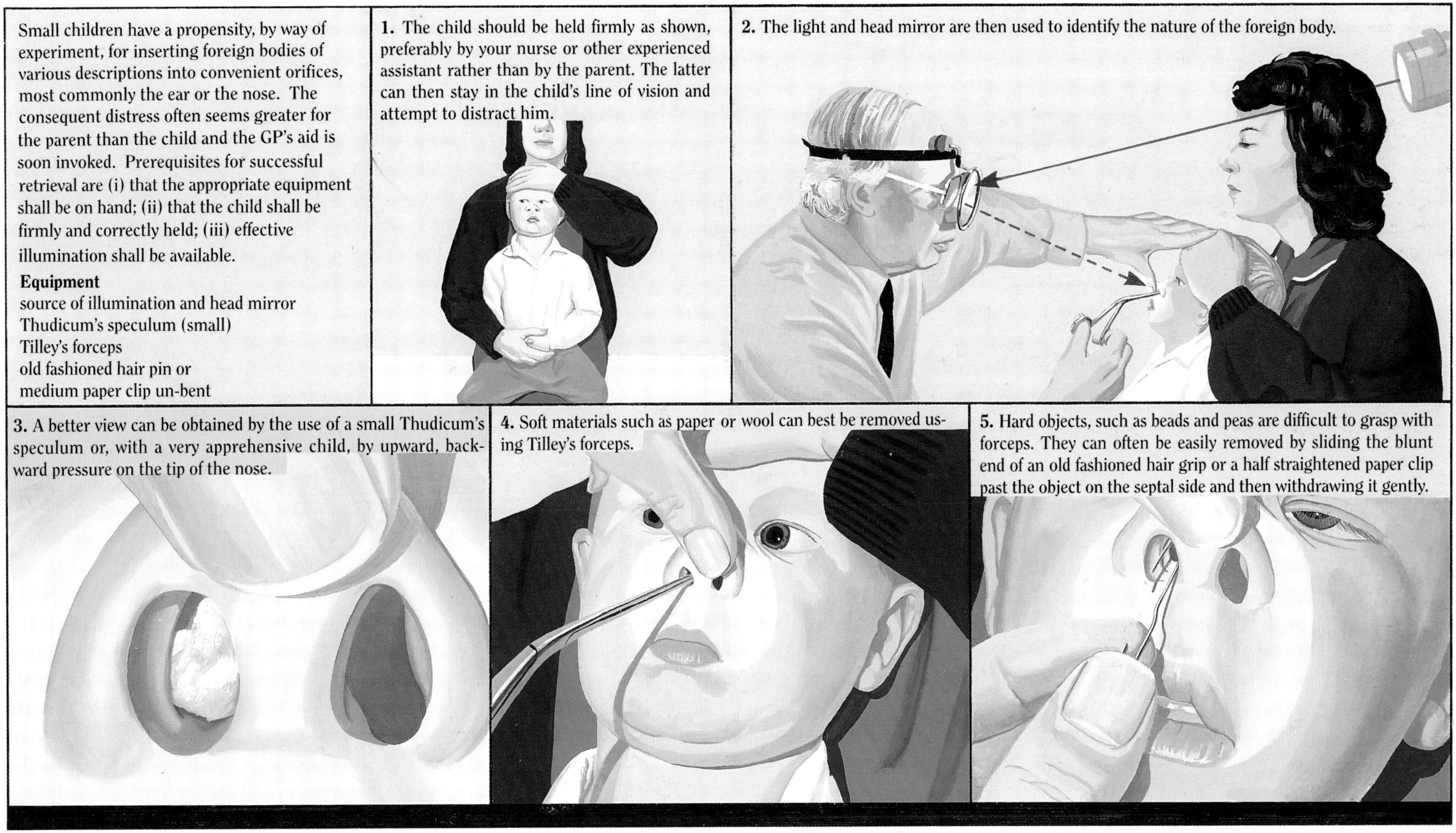

Small children have a propensity, by way of experiment, for inserting foreign bodies of various descriptions into convenient orifices, most commonly the ear or the nose. The consequent distress often seems greater for the parent than the child and the GP's aid is soon invoked. Prerequisites for successful retrieval are (i) that the appropriate equipment shall be on hand; (ii) that the child shall be firmly and correctly held; (iii) effective illumination shall be available.

Equipment
source of illumination and head mirror
Thudicum's speculum (small)
Tilley's forceps
old fashioned hair pin or
medium paper clip un-bent

1. The child should be held firmly as shown, preferably by your nurse or other experienced assistant rather than by the parent. The latter can then stay in the child's line of vision and attempt to distract him.

2. The light and head mirror are then used to identify the nature of the foreign body.

3. A better view can be obtained by the use of a small Thudicum's speculum or, with a very apprehensive child, by upward, backward pressure on the tip of the nose.

4. Soft materials such as paper or wool can best be removed using Tilley's forceps.

5. Hard objects, such as beads and peas are difficult to grasp with forceps. They can often be easily removed by sliding the blunt end of an old fashioned hair grip or a half straightened paper clip past the object on the septal side and then withdrawing it gently.

Fig. 7.50. Foreign bodies in the nose.

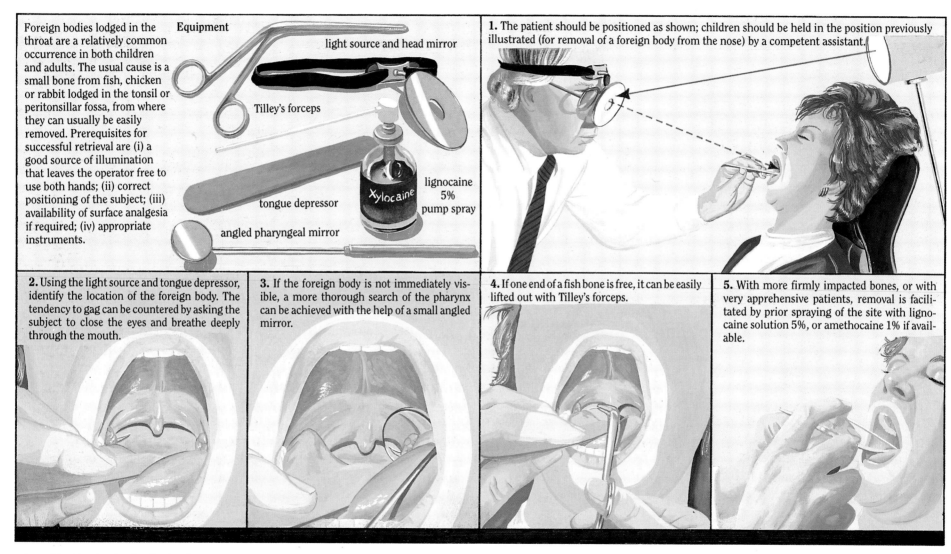

Foreign bodies lodged in the throat are a relatively common occurrence in both children and adults. The usual cause is a small bone from fish, chicken or rabbit lodged in the tonsil or peritonsillar fossa, from where they can usually be easily removed. Prerequisites for successful retrieval are (i) a good source of illumination that leaves the operator free to use both hands; (ii) correct positioning of the subject; (iii) availability of surface analgesia if required; (iv) appropriate instruments.

Equipment

light source and head mirror

Tilley's forceps

tongue depressor

Xylocaine

lignocaine 5% pump spray

angled pharyngeal mirror

1. The patient should be positioned as shown; children should be held in the position previously illustrated (for removal of a foreign body from the nose) by a competent assistant.

2. Using the light source and tongue depressor, identify the location of the foreign body. The tendency to gag can be countered by asking the subject to close the eyes and breathe deeply through the mouth.

3. If the foreign body is not immediately visible, a more thorough search of the pharynx can be achieved with the help of a small angled mirror.

4. If one end of a fish bone is free, it can be easily lifted out with Tilley's forceps.

5. With more firmly impacted bones, or with very apprehensive patients, removal is facilitated by prior spraying of the site with lignocaine solution 5%, or amethocaine 1% if available.

Fig. 7.51. Foreign bodies in the throat.

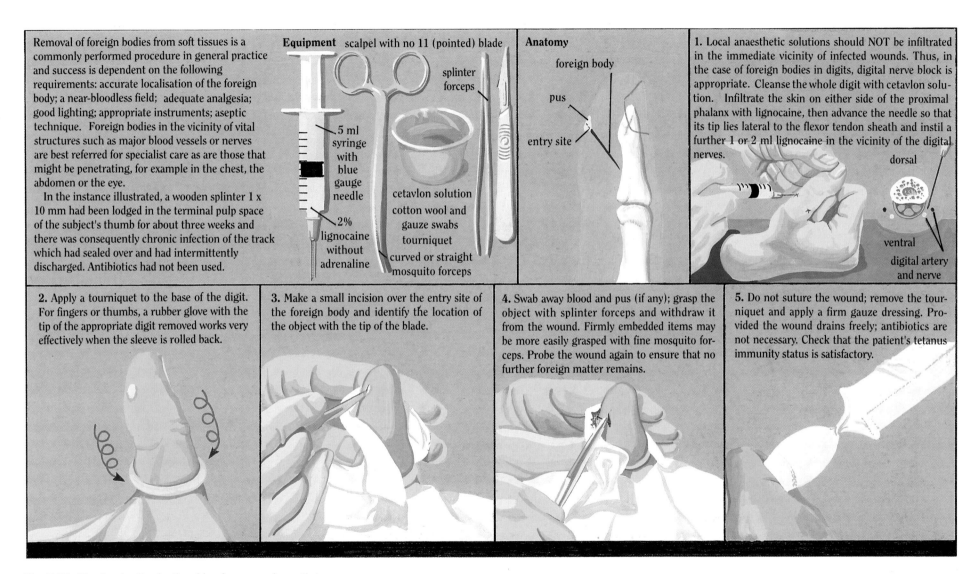

Removal of foreign bodies from soft tissues is a commonly performed procedure in general practice and success is dependent on the following requirements: accurate localisation of the foreign body; a near-bloodless field; adequate analgesia; good lighting; appropriate instruments; aseptic technique. Foreign bodies in the vicinity of vital structures such as major blood vessels or nerves are best referred for specialist care as are those that might be penetrating, for example in the chest, the abdomen or the eye.

In the instance illustrated, a wooden splinter 1 x 10 mm had been lodged in the terminal pulp space of the subject's thumb for about three weeks and there was consequently chronic infection of the track which had sealed over and had intermittently discharged. Antibiotics had not been used.

Equipment scalpel with no 11 (pointed) blade
splinter forceps
5 ml syringe with blue gauge needle
2% lignocaine without adrenaline
cetavlon solution
cotton wool and gauze swabs
tourniquet
curved or straight mosquito forceps

Anatomy
foreign body
pus
entry site

1. Local anaesthetic solutions should NOT be infiltrated in the immediate vicinity of infected wounds. Thus, in the case of foreign bodies in digits, digital nerve block is appropriate. Cleanse the whole digit with cetavlon solution. Infiltrate the skin on either side of the proximal phalanx with lignocaine, then advance the needle so that its tip lies lateral to the flexor tendon sheath and instil a further 1 or 2 ml lignocaine in the vicinity of the digital nerves.

dorsal
ventral
digital artery and nerve

2. Apply a tourniquet to the base of the digit. For fingers or thumbs, a rubber glove with the tip of the appropriate digit removed works very effectively when the sleeve is rolled back.

3. Make a small incision over the entry site of the foreign body and identify the location of the object with the tip of the blade.

4. Swab away blood and pus (if any); grasp the object with splinter forceps and withdraw it from the wound. Firmly embedded items may be more easily grasped with fine mosquito forceps. Probe the wound again to ensure that no further foreign matter remains.

5. Do not suture the wound; remove the tourniquet and apply a firm gauze dressing. Provided the wound drains freely; antibiotics are not necessary. Check that the patient's tetanus immunity status is satisfactory.

Fig. 7.52. Foreign bodies in the skin, for example, splinter.

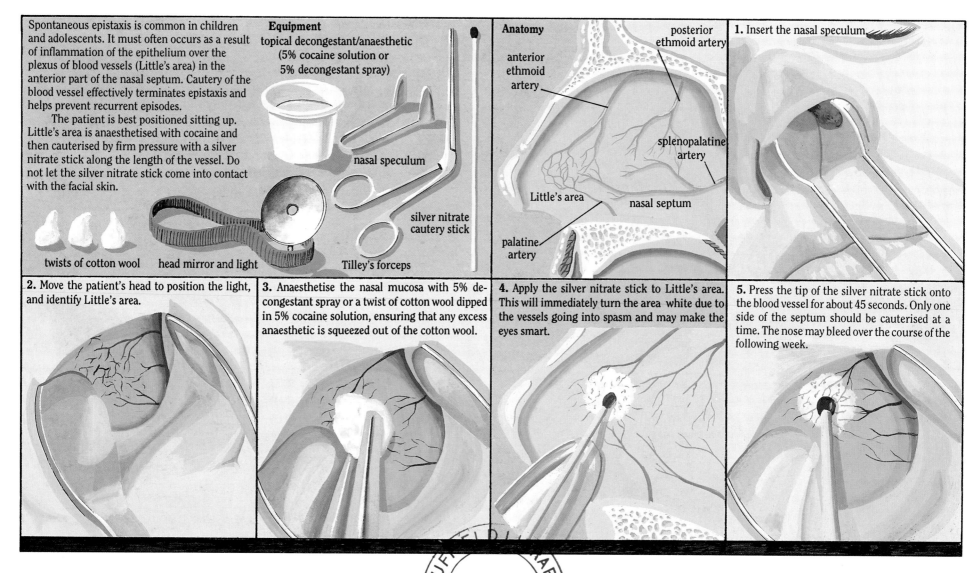

Spontaneous epistaxis is common in children and adolescents. It must often occurs as a result of inflammation of the epithelium over the plexus of blood vessels (Little's area) in the anterior part of the nasal septum. Cautery of the blood vessel effectively terminates epistaxis and helps prevent recurrent episodes.

The patient is best positioned sitting up. Little's area is anaesthetised with cocaine and then cauterised by firm pressure with a silver nitrate stick along the length of the vessel. Do not let the silver nitrate stick come into contact with the facial skin.

twists of cotton wool   head mirror and light

Equipment
topical decongestant/anaesthetic (5% cocaine solution or 5% decongestant spray)

nasal speculum

silver nitrate cautery stick

Tilley's forceps

Anatomy

anterior ethmoid artery

posterior ethmoid artery

splenopalatine artery

Little's area   nasal septum

palatine artery

1. Insert the nasal speculum.

2. Move the patient's head to position the light, and identify Little's area.

3. Anaesthetise the nasal mucosa with 5% decongestant spray or a twist of cotton wool dipped in 5% cocaine solution, ensuring that any excess anaesthetic is squeezed out of the cotton wool.

4. Apply the silver nitrate stick to Little's area. This will immediately turn the area white due to the vessels going into spasm and may make the eyes smart.

5. Press the tip of the silver nitrate stick onto the blood vessel for about 45 seconds. Only one side of the septum should be cauterised at a time. The nose may bleed over the course of the following week.

Fig. 7.53. Epistaxis: nasal cautery.

Index